Florence Nightingale

NOTES ON NURSING

フロレンス・ナイチンゲール
原文 看護覚え書

Compiled by

Hiroko Usui / Yoshihiko Kominami

原文看護学選集 1

Gendaisha Publishing Co., Ltd.
Tokyo

現 代 社

Copy from:

Florence Nightingale.
NOTES ON NURSING:
 What it is, and what it is not.
New edition, revised and
enlarged. 1860.

ナイチンゲールの原典にふれることのおすすめ

　今私たちの眼の前には、看護の長い歴史のなかにあらわれた偉大な先達、ナイチンゲールの驚嘆すべき認識を表現した数々の原典がある。私はこれまであまり読まれてこなかったこの原典を、一人でも多くの看護婦に、生のまま読んでほしいと心からねがっている。みずからの経験からたぐりとってきた彼女の論理は鋭く看護の本質をとらえており、読む人の心を激しくゆさぶるにちがいない。私は、彼女の原典が、私だけでなく、私の学生たちにも深い感動を与え、彼女たちの実習へのとりくみを一変させた事実をも見てきている。卒業をひかえた看護学生たちが、彼女の明快な文章を読み、看護を実践するよりどころをつかみとることができれば、看護婦としての成長がよりはやくなるにちがいないと思う。

　優れた実践が、優れた看護婦の長い試行錯誤の時を経てやっとたどりつけるものであってはあまりにも残念である。経験のなかにひそむ論理を探し出してくるということは、口でいうほど簡単なことではない。しかし、私たちはそれを一からはじめる必要はないのである。ナイチンゲールの認識を追体験することができれば、それを実際に使ってみることによって有効性の有無をみずから確かめることができる。

　彼女の原典にふれることの利点をもう一つ付け加えておきたい。それは、原文で読む立場が著者の認識をつかむために有効だという理由による。自国語で読む場合には、表現形式の気安さから何となくわかったつもりになることがよくある。外国語の場合には"どういう意味か？""何を言おうとしているのか？"と、いやおうなしに著者の認識をつかみとる立場に立たされるのである。彼女が発見し創り出した看護の理論を科学的な理論にしあげることは、後輩としての私たちの任務である。できるだけ多くの人々の力強いとりくみを期待したい。

　　　　　　　　　　　　1974年7月　　薄井　坦子

PREFACE

1   The following notes are by no means intended as a rule of thought by which nurses can teach themselves to nurse, still less as a manual to teach nurses to nurse. They are meant simply to give hints for thought to women who have personal charge of the health of others. Every woman, or at least almost every woman, in England has, at one time or another of her life, charge of the personal health of somebody, whether child or invalid,—in other words, every woman is a nurse. Every day sanitary knowledge, or the knowledge of nursing, or in other words, of how to put the constitution in such a state as that it will have no disease, or that it can recover from disease, takes a higher place. It is recognized as the knowledge which every one ought to have—distinct from medical knowledge, which only a profession can have.

2   If, then, every woman must, at some time or other of her life, become a nurse, *i.e.*, have charge of somebody's health, how immense and how valuable would be the produce of her united experience if every woman would think how to nurse.

3   I do not pretend to teach her how, I ask her to teach herself, and for this purpose I venture to give her some hints.

CONTENTS

Introductory 1
I. Ventilation and Warming 7
II. Health of Houses 21
III. Petty Management 33
IV. Noise 43
V. Variety 55
VI. Taking Food 61
VII. What Food? 67
VIII. Bed and Bedding 75
IX. Light 81
X. Cleanliness of Rooms and Walls 85
XI. Personal Cleanliness 91
XII. Chattering Hopes and Advices 95
XIII. Observation of the Sick 103
Conclusion 123
Supplementary Chapter 131
[Appendix] Minding Baby 153

Interpretation 159

Florence Nightingale

NOTES ON NURSING:

What it is, and what it is not.

NOTES ON NURSING:

What it is, and what it is not.

1 Shall we begin by taking it as a general principle—that all disease, at some period or other of its course, is more or less a reparative process, not necessarily accompanied with suffering: an effort of nature to remedy a process of poisoning or of decay, which has taken place weeks, months, sometimes years beforehand, unnoticed, the termination of the disease being then, while the antecedent process was going on, determined? *Disease a reparative process.*

2 If we accept this as a general principle we shall be immediately met with anecdotes and instances to prove the contrary. Just so if we were to take, as a principle—all the climates of the earth are meant to be made habitable for man, by the efforts of man—the objection would be immediately raised,—Will the top of Mont Blanc ever be made habitable? Our answer would be, it will be many thousands of years before we have reached the bottom of Mont Blanc in making the earth healthy. Wait till we have reached the bottom before we discuss the top.

3 In watching disease, both in private houses and in public hospitals, the thing which strikes the experienced observer most forcibly is *Of the suffering of disease, disease not always the cause.*

2 Introductory

this, that the symptoms or the sufferings generally considered to be inevitable and incident to the disease are very often not symptoms of the disease at all, but of something quite different—of the want of fresh air, or of light, or of warmth, or of quiet, or of cleanliness, or of punctuality and care in the administration of diet, of each or of all of these. And this quite as much in private as in hospital nursing.

4 The reparative process which Nature has instituted, and which we call disease, has been hindered by some want of knowledge or attention, in one or in all of these things, and pain, suffering, or interruption of the whole process sets in.

5 If a patient is cold, if a patient is feverish, if a patient is faint, if he is sick after taking food, if he has a bed-sore, it is generally the fault not of the disease, but of the nursing.

What nursing ought to do.

6 I use the word nursing for want of a better. It has been limited to signify little more than the administration of medicines and the application of poultices. It ought to signify the proper use of fresh air, light, warmth, cleanliness, quiet, and the proper selection and administration of diet—all at the least expense of vital power to the patient.

Nursing the sick little understood.

7 It has been said and written scores of times, that every woman makes a good nurse. I believe, on the contrary, that the very elements of nursing are all but unknown.

8 By this I do not mean that the nurse is always to blame. Bad sanitary, bad architectural, and bad administrative arrangements often make it impossible to nurse. But the art of nursing ought to include such arrangements as alone make what I understand by nursing possible.

Nursing ought to assist the reparative process.

9 To recur to the first objection. If we are asked, Is such or such a disease a reparative process? Can such an illness be unaccompanied with suffering? Will any care prevent such a patient from suffering this or that?—I humbly say, I do not know. But when you have done away with all that pain and suffering, which in patients are the symptoms not of their disease, but of the absence of one or all of the above-mentioned essentials to the success of Nature's reparative processes, we shall then know what are the symptoms of and the sufferings inseparable from the disease.

10 Another and the commonest exclamation which will be instantly made is—Would you do nothing, then, in cholera, fever, &c.?—so deep-

rooted and universal is the conviction that to give medicine is to be doing something, or rather everything; to give air, warmth, cleanliness, &c., is to do nothing. The reply is, that in these and many other similar diseases the exact value of particular remedies and modes of treatment is by no means ascertained, while there is universal experience as to the extreme importance of careful nursing in determining the issue of the disease.

11   II. The very elements of what constitutes good nursing are as little understood for the well as for the sick. The same laws of health or of nursing, for they are in reality the same, obtain among the well as among the sick. The breaking of them produces only a less violent consequence among the former than among the latter,—and this sometimes, not always. *Nursing the well*

12   It is constantly objected,—"But how can I obtain this medical knowledge? I am not a doctor. I must leave this to doctors."

13   Oh, mothers of families! You who say this, do you know that one in every seven infants in this civilized land of England perishes before it is one year old? That, in London, two in every five die before they are five years old? And, in the other great cities of England, nearly one out of two? *Little understood.*

14   Upon this fact the most wonderful deductions have been strung. For a long time an announcement something like the following has been going the round of the papers:—"More than 25,000 children die every year in London under 10 years of age; therefore we want a Children's Hospital." Last spring there was a prospectus issued, and divers other means taken to this effect:—"There is a great want of sanitary knowledge in women; therefore we want a Women's Hospital." Now, both the above facts are too sadly true. But what is the deduction? The causes of the enormous child mortality are perfectly well known; they are chiefly want of cleanliness, want of ventilation, careless dieting and clothing, want of white-washing; in one word, defective *household* hygiene. The remedies are just as well known; and among them is certainly not the establishment of a Child's Hospital. This may be a want; just as there may be a want of hospital room for adults. But the Registrar-General would certainly never think of giving us, as a cause for the high rate of child mortality in (say) Liverpool, that there was not sufficient hospital room for children; nor would he urge upon us, as a remedy, to found a hospital *Curious deductions from an excessive death rate.*

4 Introductory

for them.

15 Again, women, and the best women, are woefully deficient in sanitary knowledge; although it is to women that we must look, first and last, for its application, as far as *household* hygiene is concerned. But who would ever think of citing the institution of a Women's Hospital as the way to cure this want?

16 We have it, indeed, upon very high authority that there is some fear lest hospitals, as they have been *hitherto,* may not have generally increased, rather than diminished, the rate of mortality—especially of child mortality.

<small>Child life a test of healthy conditions.</small>

17 "The life duration of tender babies" (as some Saturn, turned analytical chemist, says) "is the most delicate test" of sanitary conditions. Is all this premature suffering and death necessary? Or did Nature intend mothers to be always accompanied by doctors? Or is it better to learn the piano-forte than to learn the laws which subserve the preservation of offspring?

18 Macaulay somewhere says, that it is extraordinary that, whereas the laws of the motions of the heavenly bodies, far removed as they are from us, are perfectly well understood, the laws of the human mind, which are under our observation all day and every day, are no better understood than they were two thousand years ago.

19 But how much more extraordinary is it that, whereas what we might call the coxcombries of education—*e.g.,* the elements of astronomy—are now taught to every school-girl, neither mothers of families of any class, nor school-mistresses of any class, nor nurses of children, nor nurses of hospitals, are taught anything about those laws which God has assigned to the relations of our bodies with the world in which He has put them. In other words, the laws which make these bodies, into which He has put our minds, healthy or unhealthy organs of those minds, are all but unlearnt. Not but that these laws—the laws of life—are in a certain measure understood, but not even mothers think it worth their while to study them—to study how to give their children healthy existences. They call it medical or physiological knowledge, fit only for doctors.

20 Another objection.

21 We are constantly told,—"But the circumstances which govern our children's healths are beyond our control. What can we do with winds? There is the east wind. Most people can tell before they get up in the

morning whether the wind is in the east."

22   To this one can answer with more certainty than to the former objections. Who is it who knows when the wind is in the east? Not the Highland drover, certainly, exposed to the east wind, but the young lady who is worn out with the want of exposure to fresh air, to sunlight, &c. Put the latter under as good sanitary circumstances as the former, and she too will not know when the wind is in the east.

I. VENTILATION AND WARMING.

1   The very first canon of nursing, the first and the last thing upon which a nurse's attention must be fixed, the first essential to the patient, without which all the rest you can do for him is as nothing, with which I had almost said you may leave all the rest alone, is this: To keep the air he breathes as pure as the external air, without chilling him. Yet what is so little attended to? Even where it is thought of at all, the most extraordinary misconceptions reign about it. Even in admitting air into the patient's room or ward, few people ever think where that air comes from. It may come from a corridor into which other wards are ventilated, from a hall, always unaired, always full of the fumes of gas, dinner, of various kinds of mustiness; from an underground kitchen, sink, wash-house, water-closet, or even, as I myself have had sorrowful experience, from open sewers loaded with filth; and with this the patient's room or ward is aired, as it is called—poisoned, it should rather be said. Always air from the air without, and that, too, through those windows, through which the air comes freshest. From a closed court, especially if the wind do not blow that way, air may come as stagnant as any from a hall or corridor.

First rule of nursing, to keep the air within as pure as the air without.

2   Again, a thing I have often seen both in private houses and institutions. A room remains uninhabited; the fire-place is carefully fastened up with a board; the windows are never opened; probably the shutters are kept always shut; perhaps some kind of stores are

Ventilation & Warming

kept in the room: no breath of fresh air can by possibility enter into that room, nor any ray of sun. The air is as stagnant, musty, and corrupt as it can by possibility be made. It is quite ripe to breed small-pox, scarlet fever, diphtheria, or anything else you please.

3   Yet the nursery, ward, or sick room adjoining will positively be aired (?) by having the door opened into that room. Or children will be put into that room, without previous preparation, to sleep.

Why are uninhabited rooms shut up?

4   The common idea as to uninhabited rooms is that they may safely be left with doors, windows, shutters, and chimney board, all closed —hermetically sealed if possible—to keep out the dust, it is said; and that no harm will happen if the room is but opened a short hour before the inmates are put in. The question has often been asked for uninhabited rooms—But when ought the windows to be opened? The answer is—When ought they to be shut?

A common madness.

5   A short time ago a man walked into a back-kitchen in Queen's-square, and cut the throat of a poor consumptive creature, sitting by the fire. The murderer did not deny the act, but simply said, "It's all right." Of course he was mad.

6   But in our case, the extraordinary thing is that the victim says, "It's all right," and that we are not mad. Yet, although we "nose" the murderers in the musty, unaired, unsunned room, the scarlet fever which is behind the door, or the fever and hospital gangrene which are stalking among the crowded beds of a hospital ward, we say, "It's all right."

How to ventilate without chill

7   With a proper supply of windows, and a proper supply of fuel in open fire places, fresh air is comparatively easy to secure when your patient or patients are in bed. Never be afraid of open windows then. People don't catch cold in bed. This is a popular fallacy. With proper bed-clothes and hot bottles, if necessary, you can always keep a patient warm in bed, and well ventilate him at the same time.

8   But a careless nurse, be her rank and education what it may, will stop up every cranny, and keep a hot-house heat when her patient is in bed,—and, if he is able to get up, leave him comparatively unprotected. The time when people take cold (and there are many ways of taking cold, besides a cold in the nose,) is when they first get up after the two-fold exhaustion of dressing and of having had the skin relaxed by many hours, perhaps days, in bed, and thereby rendered more incapable of re-action. Then the same temperature which

refreshes the patient in bed may destroy the patient just risen. And common sense will point out that, while purity of air is essential, a temperature must be secured which shall not chill the patient. Otherwise, the best that can be expected will be a feverish reaction.

9   To have the air within as pure as the air without, it is not necessary, as often appears to be thought, to make it as cold.

10   In the afternoon again, without care, the patient whose vital powers have then risen often finds the room as close and oppressive as he found it cold in the morning. Yet the nurse will be terrified if a window is opened.

11   It is very desirable that the windows in a sick room should be such as that the patient shall, if he can move about, be able to open and shut them easily himself.* In fact, the sick room is very seldom kept aired if this is not the case—so very few people have any perception of what is a healthy atmosphere for the sick. The sick man often says, "This room, where I spend twenty-two hours out of the twenty-four is fresher than the other where I only spend two. Because here I can manage the windows myself." And it is true.

12   I know an intelligent humane house surgeon who makes a practice of keeping the ward windows open. The physicians and surgeons invariably close them while going their rounds; and the house surgeon, very properly, as invariably opens them whenever the doctors have turned their backs.   *Open windows*

13   In a little book on nursing, published a short time ago, we are told, that "with proper care it is very seldom that the windows cannot be opened for a few minutes twice in the day to admit fresh air from without." I should think not; nor twice in the hour either. It only shows how little the subject has been considered.

14   Of all methods of keeping patients warm the very worst certainly is to depend for heat on the breath and bodies of the sick. I have known a medical officer keep his ward windows hermetically closed, thus exposing the sick to all the dangers of an infected atmosphere, because he was afraid that, by admitting fresh air, the temperature   *What kind of warmth desirable.*

(11)   * Note.—Delirious fever cases, where there is any danger of the patient jumping out of window, are, of course, exceptions. It is absolutely necessary that such cases should be kept cool and well aired. I would undertake, with four gimlets, to save all risk of accidents, by merely preventing the sashes, both upper and lower, from being opened more than a few inches.

10 Ventilation & Warming

of the ward would be too much lowered. This is a destructive fallacy.

15   To attempt to keep a ward warm at the expense of making the sick repeatedly breathe their own hot, humid, putrescing atmosphere is a certain way to delay recovery or to destroy life.

Bedrooms almost universally foul.

16   Do you ever go into the bed-rooms of any persons of any class, whether they contain one, two, or twenty people, whether they hold sick or well, at night, or before the windows are opened in the morning, and ever find the air anything but unwholesomely close and foul? And why should it be so? And of how much importance is it that it should not be so? During sleep, the human body, even when in health, is far more injured by the influence of foul air than when awake. Why can't you keep the air all night, then, as pure as the air without in the rooms you sleep in? But for this, you must have sufficient outlet for the impure air you make yourself to go out; sufficient inlet for the pure air from without to come in. You must have open chimneys, open windows, or ventilators; no close curtains round your beds; no shutters or curtains to your windows, none of the contrivances by which you undermine your own health or destroy the chances of recovery of your sick.

How to open your windows.

17   Open the window above, not below. If your windows do not open above, the sooner they are made to do so the better. An inch or two will be enough for two people in a moderately-sized bedroom in winter. In a children's nursery or bedroom more will be required, according to the number. The worst place to admit air either into sick room or hospital ward, is at or near the level of the floor. Air admitted in this situation cools the floor and the lower strata of air; and if the patient is able to step out of bed, the cold air may give him a dangerous chill. During mild weather and summer time your windows may be wide open. In this, as in other things, common sense must be used. Ventilation of a bedroom or a sick room does not mean throwing the window up to the top, or drawing it down as far as it will come; still less does it mean opening the windows at intervals and keeping them shut between times, thereby subjecting the patient to the risk of frequent and violent alternations of temperature. It means simply keeping the air fresh.

18   The true criterion of this is to step out of the bedroom or sick room, in the morning, into the open air. If, on returning to it, you feel the least sensation of closeness, the ventilation has not been enough,

and that room has been unfit for either sick or well to sleep in.

19   Of all places, public or private schools, where a number of children or young persons sleep in the same dormitory, require this test of freshness to be constantly applied. If it be hazardous for two children to sleep together in an unventilated bedroom, it is more than doubly so to have four, and much more than trebly so to have six under the same circumstances. People rarely remember this; yet, if parents were as solicitous about the air of school bedrooms as they are about the food the children are to eat, and the kind of education they are to receive, at school, depend upon it due attention would be bestowed on this vitally important matter, and they would cease to have their children sent home either ill, or because scarlet fever or some other "current contagion" had broken out in the school. There are schools where attention is paid to these things, and where "children's epidemics" are unknown.   *Schools.*

20   How much sickness, death, and misery are produced by the present state of many factories, warehouses, workshops, and workrooms! The places where poor dressmakers, tailors, letter-press printers, and other similar trades have to work for their living, are generally in a worse sanitary condition than any other portion of our worst towns. Many of these places of work were never constructed for such an object. They are badly adapted garrets, sitting-rooms, or bedrooms, generally of an inferior class of house. No attention is paid to cubic space or ventilation. The poor workers are crowded on the floor to a greater extent than occurs with any other kind of overcrowding. In many cases 100 cubic feet would be considered by employers an extravagant extent of space for a worker. The constant breathing of foul air, saturated with moisture, and the action of such air upon the skin renders the inmates peculiarly susceptible of the impression of cold, which is an index indeed of the danger of pulmonary disease to which they are exposed. The result is, that they make bad worse, by over-heating the air and closing up every cranny through which ventilation could be obtained. In such places, and under such circumstances of constrained posture, want of exercise, hurried and insufficient meals, long exhausting labour and foul air —is it wonderful that a great majority of them die early of chest disease, generally of consumption? Intemperance is a common evil of these workshops. The men can only complete their work under   *Work-rooms.*

12 Ventilation & Warming

the influence of stimulants, which help to undermine their health and destroy their morals, while hurrying them to premature graves. Employers rarely consider these things. Healthy workrooms are no part of the bond into which they enter with their work-people. They pay their money, which they reckon their part of the bargain. And for this wage the workman or workwoman has to give work, health, and life.

21   Do men and women who employ fashionable tailors and milliners ever think of these things?

An air-test of essential consequence.

22   And yet the master is no gainer. His goods are spoiled by foul air and gas fumes, his own health and that of his family suffers, and his work is not so well done as it would be, were his people in health. It is now admitted to be cheaper for all manufacturing purposes to have pure soft water than hard water. And the time will come when it will be found cheaper to supply shops, warehouses, and workrooms with pure air than with foul air.

23   Dr. Angus Smith's air-test, if it could be made of simple application, would be invaluable to use in every sleeping and sick room. Just as without the use of a thermometer no nurse should ever put a patient into a bath, so, if this air-test were made in some equally simple form, should no nurse, or mother, or superintendent, be without it in any ward, nursery, or sleeping-room. But to be used, the air-test must be made as simple a little instrument as the thermometer, and both should be self-registering. The senses of nurses and mothers become so dulled to foul air that they are perfectly unconscious of what an atmosphere they have let their children, patients, or charges sleep in. But if the tell-tale air-test were to exhibit in the morning, both to nurses and patient and to the superior officer going round, what the atmosphere has been during the night, I question if any greater security could be afforded against a recurrence of the misdemeanour.

24   And, oh! the crowded national school! where so many children's epidemics have their origin; and the crowded, unventilated workroom, which sends so many consumptive men and women to the grave; what a tale its air-test would tell! We should have parents saying, and saying rightly, "I will not send my child to that school. I will not trust my son or my daughter in that tailor's or milliner's workshop, the air-test stands at 'Horrid.'" And the dormitories of our

great boarding schools! Scarlet fever would be no more ascribed to contagion but to its right cause, the air-test standing at "Foul."

25 We should hear no longer of "mysterious dispensations," nor of "plague and pestilence" being "in God's hands," when, so far as we know, He has put them into our own. The little air-test would both betray the cause of these "mysterious pestilences," and call upon us to remedy it.

26 A careful nurse will keep a constant watch over her sick, especially weak, protracted, and collapsed cases, to guard against the effects of the loss of vital heat by the patient himself. In certain diseased states much less heat is produced than in health; and there is a constant tendency to the decline and ultimate extinction of the vital powers by the call made upon them to sustain the heat of the body. Cases where this occurs should be watched with the greatest care from hour to hour, I had almost said from minute to minute. The feet and legs should be examined by the hand from time to time, and whenever a tendency to chilling is discovered, hot bottles, hot bricks, or warm flannels, with some warm drink, should be made use of until the temperature is restored. The fire should be, if necessary, replenished. Patients are frequently lost in the latter stages of disease from want of attention to such simple precautions. The nurse may be trusting to the patient's diet, or to his medicine, or to the occasional dose of stimulant which she is directed to give him, while the patient is all the while sinking from want of a little external warmth. Such cases happen at all times, even during the height of summer. This fatal chill is most apt to occur towards early morning at the period of the lowest temperature of the twenty-four hours, and at the time when the effect of the preceding day's diets is exhausted.
_{When warmth must be most carefully looked to.}

27 Generally speaking, you may expect that weak patients will suffer cold much more in the morning than in the evening. The vital powers are much lower. If they are feverish at night, with burning hands and feet, they are almost sure to be chilly and shivering in the morning. But nurses are very fond of heating the foot-warmer at night, and of neglecting it in the morning, when they are busy. I should reverse the matter.

28 What can nurses be thinking of who put a bottle of boiling water to the patient's feet, hoping that it will keep warm all the twenty-four hours ? Of course, every time he touches it, it wakes him. It sends
_{Hot bottles.}

14 Ventilation & Warming

the blood to the head. It makes his feet tender. And then the nurse leaves it in the bed after it has become quite cold. A hot bottle should never be hotter than it can be comfortably touched with the naked hand. It should not be expected to keep warm longer than eight hours. Tin foot-warmers are too hot and too cold. Stone bottles are the best, or India-rubber. But careless nurses make sad havoc with the latter, by putting in water too hot, or by letting the screw get out of order, and the patient be deluged in his bed.

29   All these things require common sense and care. Yet perhaps in no one single thing is so little common sense shown, in all ranks, as in nursing.

30   The art of nursing, as now practised, seems to be expressly constituted to unmake what God had made disease to be, viz., a reparative process.

Cold air not ventilation, nor fresh air a method of chill.

31   The extraordinary confusion between cold and ventilation, in the minds of even well educated people, illustrates this. To make a room cold is by no means necessarily to ventilate it. Nor is it at all necessary, in order to ventilate a room, to chill it. Yet, if a nurse finds a room close, she will let out the fire, thereby making it closer, or she will open the door into a cold room, without a fire, or an open window in it, by way of improving the ventilation. The safest atmosphere of all for a patient is a good fire and an open window, excepting in extremes of temperature. (Yet no nurse can ever be made to understand this.) To ventilate a small room without draughts of course requires more care than to ventilate a large one.

32   With private sick, I think, but certainly with hospital sick, the nurse should never be satisfied as to the freshness of their atmosphere, unless she can feel the air gently moving over her face, when still.

Draughts.

33   But it is often observed that nurses who make the greatest outcry against open windows are those who take the least pains to prevent dangerous draughts. The door of the patients' room or ward *must* sometimes **stand** open to allow of persons passing in and out, or heavy things being carried in and out. The careful nurse will keep the door shut while she shuts the windows, and then, and not before, set the door open, so that a patient may not be left sitting up in bed, perhaps in a profuse perspiration, directly in the draught between the open door and window. Neither, of course, should a patient, while

being washed or in any way exposed, remain in the draught of an open window or door.

34 It is truly provoking to see stupid women bring into disrepute the life-spring of the patient, viz., fresh air, by their stupidity. Chest and throat attacks may undoubtedly be brought on by the nurse letting her sick run about without slippers, flannel or dressing-gowns, in a room where she has left the wintry wind blowing in upon them, without taking any precaution if they should leave their beds. Certain beds are sometimes pointed out in certain wards, in a kind of helpless way, as being predestined to bronchitis, because of the "draught from the door." Why should there be a draught from the door? If there be, why should the draught fall on a patient? Is there no such thing as a screen to be had; or if the bed space be in a draught which cannot be prevented, why not remove the bed? The same thing happens frequently in private sick rooms. A careless nurse will leave a window open on one side of a patient, and a door on the other. It never seems to occur to her that window-sashes can be put down while there is occasion for opening the door. She will come into the sick room and leave the door open till she goes out again, for no reason that any body can discover but her own blindness. And she will leave the window open over her patient who is washing or sitting up in a night-dress, and then say, "He has taken cold from the open window." He has taken cold from your own thoughtlessness. Neither leaving doors open nor drawing down windows over your patients when the surface is exposed is ventilation. It is simply carelessness.

35 Another extraordinary fallacy is the dread of night air. What air can we breathe at night but night air? The choice is between pure night air from without, and foul night air from within. Most people prefer the latter. An unaccountable choice. What will they say if it is proved to be true that fully one-half of all the disease we suffer from is occasioned by people sleeping with their windows shut? An open window most nights in the year can never hurt any one. This is not to say that light is not necessary for recovery. In great cities, night air is often the best and purest air to be had in the twenty-four hours. I could better understand in towns shutting the windows during the day than during the night, for the sake of the sick. The absence of smoke, the quiet, all tend to making night the best time for airing the patients. One of our highest medical authorities on Con-

Night air.

16 Ventilation & Warming

sumption and Climate has told me that the air in London is never so good as after ten o'clock at night.

36 The only time when it can be unsafe to open the window at night is when the air is more foul without than within. This may be the case in close back courts, and in malarial countries, or at hours when there is a sudden fall of temperature. But even in malarial districts it is found that thin gauze curtains, while admitting the air, are a protection from malaria.

Air from the outside. Open your windows, shut your doors.

37 Always air your room, then, from the outside air, if possible. Windows are made to open; doors are made to shut—a truth which seems extremely difficult of apprehension. I have seen a careful nurse airing her patient's room through the door near to which were two gaslights (each of which consumes as much air as eleven men), a kitchen, a corridor, the composition of the atmosphere in which consisted of gas, paint, foul air, never changed, full of effluvia, including a current of sewer air from an ill-placed sink, ascending in a continual stream by a well-staircase and discharging themselves constantly into the patient's room. The window of the said room, if opened, was all that was desirable to air it. Every room must be aired from without—every passage from without—But the fewer passages there are in a hospital the better.

Smoke.

38 If we are to preserve the air within as pure as the air without, it is needless to say that the chimney must not smoke. Almost all smoky chimneys can be cured—from the bottom, not from the top. Often it is only necessary to have an inlet for air to supply the fire, which is feeding itself, for want of this, from its own chimney. On the other hand, almost all chimneys can be made to smoke by a careless nurse, who lets the fire get low, and then overwhelms it with coal; not, as we verily believe, in order to spare herself trouble (for very rare is unkindness to the sick), but from not thinking what she is about.

Airing damp things in a patient's room.

39 In laying down the principle that the first object of the nurse must be to keep the air breathed by her patient as pure as the air without, it must not be forgotten that everything in the room which can give off effluvia, besides the patient, evaporates itself into his air. And it follows that there ought to be nothing in the room, excepting him, which can give off effluvia or moisture. Out of all damp towels, &c., which become dry in the room, the damp, of course, goes into the

patient's air. Yet this "of course" seems as little thought of as if it were an obsolete fiction. How very seldom you see a nurse who acknowledges by her practice that nothing at all ought to be aired in the patient's room, that nothing at all ought to be cooked at the patient's fire! Indeed the arrangements often make this rule impossible to observe.

40   If the nurse be a very careful one, she will, when the patient leaves his bed, but not his room, open the sheets wide, and throw the bed clothes back, in order to air his bed. And she will spread the wet towels or flannels carefully out upon a horse, in order to dry them. Now either these bed clothes and towels are not dried and aired, or they dry and air themselves into the patient's air. And whether the damp and effluvia do him most harm in his air or in his bed, I leave to you to determine, for I cannot.

41   Even in health people cannot repeatedly breathe air in which they live with impunity, on account of its becoming charged with unwholesome matter from the lungs and skin. In disease, where everything given off from the body is highly noxious and dangerous, not only must there be plenty of ventilation to carry off the effluvia, but everything which the patient passes must be instantly removed away, as being more noxious than even the emanations from the sick. *Effluvia from excreta.*

42   Of the fatal effects of the effluvia from the excreta it would seem unnecessary to speak, were they not so constantly neglected. Concealing the utensil behind the vallance to the bed seems all the precaution which is thought necessary for safety in private nursing. Did you but think for one moment of the atmosphere under that bed, the saturation of the under side of the mattress with the warm evaporations, you would be startled and frightened too!

43   The use of any chamber utensil *without a lid* should be utterly abolished, whether among sick or well. You can easily convince yourself of the necessity of this absolute rule, by taking one with a lid, and examining the under side of that lid. It will be found always covered, whenever the utensil is not empty, by condensed offensive moisture. Where does that go, when there is no lid? *Chamber utensils without lids.*

44   But never, never should the possession of this indispensable lid confirm you in the abominable practice of letting the chamber utensil remain in a patient's room unemptied, except once in the twenty-four hours, *i.e.,* when the bed is made. Yes, impossible as it may appear, *Don't make your sick-room into a sewer.*

18 Ventilation & Warming

I have known the best and most attentive nurses guilty of this; aye, and have known, too, a patient afflicted with severe diarrhœa for ten days, and the nurse (a very good one) not know of it, because the chamber utensil (one with a lid) was emptied only once in the twenty-four hours, and that by the housemaid who came in and made the patient's bed every evening. As well might you have a sewer under the room, or think that in a water-closet the plug need be pulled up but once a day. Also take care that your lid, as well as your utensil, be always thoroughly rinsed.

45   If a nurse declines to do these kinds of things for her patient, "because it is not her business," I should say that nursing was not her calling. I have seen surgical "sisters," women whose hands were worth to them two or three guineas a-week, down upon their knees scouring a room or hut, because they thought it otherwise not fit for their patients to go into. I am far from wishing nurses to scour. It is a waste of power. But I do say that these women had the true nurse-calling—the good of their sick first, and second only the consideration what it was their "place" to do—and that women who wait for the housemaid to do this, or for the charwoman to do that, when their patients are suffering, have not the *making* of a nurse in them.

46   Earthenware, or if there is any wood, highly polished and varnished wood, are the only materials fit for patients' utensils. The very lid of the old abominable close-stool is enough to breed a pestilence. It becomes saturated with offensive matter, which scouring is only wanted to bring out. I prefer an earthenware lid as being always cleaner. But there are various good new-fashioned arrangements.

Abolish slop-pails. 47   A slop-pail should never be brought into a sick room. It should be a rule invariable, rather more important in the private house than elsewhere, that the utensil should be carried directly to the water-closet, emptied there, rinsed there, and brought back. There should always be water and a cock in every water-closet for rinsing. But even if there is not, you must carry water there to rinse with. I have actually seen, in the private sick room, the utensils emptied into the foot-pan, and put back, unrinsed, under the bed. I can hardly say which is most abominable, whether to do this or to rinse the utensil *in* the sick room. In the best hospitals it is now a rule that no slop-pail shall ever be brought into the wards, but that the utensils shall be carried direct to be emptied and rinsed at the proper place. I would it were so in the private house.

48   Let no one ever depend upon fumigations, "disinfectants," and the like, for purifying the air. The offensive thing, not its smell, must be removed. A celebrated medical lecturer began one day, "Fumigations, gentlemen, are of essential importance. They make such an abominable smell that they compel you to open the window." I wish all disinfecting fluids invented made such an "abominable smell" that they forced you to admit fresh air. That would be a useful invention.   Fumigations.

II. HEALTH OF HOUSES.*

1   There are five essential points in securing the health of houses:—

        1. Pure air.
        2. Pure water.
        3. Efficient drainage.
        4. Cleanliness.
        5. Light.

[margin: Health of houses. Five points essential.]

Without these, no house can be healthy. And it will be unhealthy just in proportion as they are deficient.

2   1. To have pure air, your house must be so constructed as that the outer atmosphere shall find its way with ease to every corner of it. House architects hardly ever consider this. The object in building a house is to obtain the largest interest for the money, not to save doctor's bills to the tenants. But, if tenants should ever become so wise as to refuse to occupy unhealthily constructed houses, and if Insurance Companies should ever come to understand their interest

[margin: Pure air.]

(0')   * The health of carriages, especially close carriages, is not of sufficient universal importance to mention here, otherwise than cursorily. Children, who are always the most delicate test of sanitary conditions, generally cannot enter a close carriage without being sick—and very lucky for them that it is so. A close carriage, with the horse-hair cushions and linings always saturated with organic matter, and unaired from the musty foulness of the coach-house, if to this be added the windows up, is one of the most unhealthy of human receptacles. The idea of taking an airing in it is something preposterous. Dr. Angus Smith has shown that a crowded railway carriage, which goes at the rate of 30 miles an hour, is as unwholesome as the strong smell of a sewer, or as a back yard in one of the most unhealthy courts off one of the most unhealthy streets in Manchester.

[margin: Health of carriages.]

so thoroughly as to pay a Sanitary Surveyor to look after the houses where their clients live, speculative architects would speedily be brought to their senses. As it is, they build what pays best. And there are always people foolish enough to take the houses they build. And if in the course of time the families die off, as is so often the case, nobody ever thinks of blaming any but Providence for the result. Ill-informed medical men aid in sustaining the delusion, by laying the blame on "current contagions." Badly constructed houses do for the healthy what badly constructed hospitals do for the sick. Once insure that the air in a house is stagnant, and sickness is certain to follow.

<small>Pure water.</small> 3   2. Pure water is more generally introduced into houses than it used to be, thanks to the exertions of the sanitary reformers. Within the last few years, a large part of London was in the daily habit of using water polluted by the drainage of its sewers and water closets. This has happily been remedied. But, in many parts of the country, well water of a very impure kind is used for domestic purposes. And when epidemic disease shows itself, persons using such water are almost sure to suffer.

<small>Drainage.</small> 4   3. It would be curious to ascertain by inspection, how many houses in London are really well drained. Many people would say, surely all or most of them. But many people have no idea in what good drainage consists. They think that a sewer in the street, and a pipe leading to it from the house is good drainage. All the while the sewer may be nothing but a laboratory from which epidemic disease and ill health is being distilled into the house. No house with any untrapped unventilated drain pipe communicating immediately with an unventilated sewer, whether it be from water closet, sink, or gully-grate, can ever be healthy. An untrapped sink may at any time spread fever or pyæmia among the inmates of a palace.

<small>Sinks.</small> 5   The ordinary oblong sink is an abomination. That great surface of stone, which is always left wet, is always exhaling into the air. I have known whole houses and hospitals smell of the sink. I have met just as strong a stream of sewer air coming up the back staircase of a grand London house from the sink, as I have ever met at Scutari; and I have seen the rooms in that house all ventilated by the open doors, and the passages all *un*ventilated by the closed windows, in order that as much of the sewer air as possible might be conducted

into and retained in the bed-rooms. It is wonderful!

6   Another great evil in house construction is carrying drains underneath the house. Such drains are never safe. All house drains should begin and end outside the walls. Many people will readily admit, as a theory, the importance of these things. But how few are there who can intelligently trace disease in their households to such causes! Is it not a fact, that when scarlet fever, measles, or small-pox appear among the children, the very first thought which occurs is "where" the children can have "caught" the disease? And the parents immediately run over in their minds all the families with whom they may have been. They never think of looking at home for the source of the mischief. If a neighbour's child is seized with small-pox, the first question which occurs is whether it had been vaccinated. No one would undervalue vaccination; but it becomes of doubtful benefit to society when it leads people to look abroad for the source of evils which exist at home.

7   4. Without cleanliness, within and without your house, ventilation is comparatively useless. In certain foul districts of London, poor people used to object to open their windows and doors because of the foul smells that came in. Rich people like to have their stables and dunghill near their houses. But does it ever occur to them that with many arrangements of this kind it would be safer to keep the windows shut than open? You cannot have the air of the house pure with dung heaps under the windows. These are common all over London. And yet people are surprised that their children, brought up in large "well-aired" nurseries and bed-rooms suffer from children's epidemics. If they studied Nature's laws in the matter of children's health, they would not be so surprised.   _{Cleanliness.}

8   There are other ways of having filth inside a house besides having dirt in heaps. Old papered walls of years' standing, dirty carpets, uncleaned furniture, are just as ready sources of impurity to the air as if there were a dung-heap in the basement. People are so unaccustomed from education and habits to consider how to make a home healthy, that they either never think of it at all, and take every disease as a matter of course, to be "resigned to" when it comes "as from the hand of Providence;" or if they ever entertain the idea of preserving the health of their household as a duty, they are very apt to commit all kinds of "negligences and ignorances" in performing it.

24 Health of Houses

Light.

5. A dark house is always an unhealthy house, always an ill-aired house, always a dirty house. Want of light stops growth, and promotes scrofula, rickets, &c., among the children.

People lose their health in a dark house, and if they get ill they cannot get well again in it. More will be said about this farther on.

Three common errors in managing the health of houses.

Three out of many "negligences and ignorances" in managing the health of houses generally, I will here mention as specimens—
1. That the female head in charge of any building does not think it necessary to visit every hole and corner of it every day. How can she expect those who are under her to be more careful to maintain her house in a healthy condition than she who is in charge of it?—
2. That it is not considered essential to air, to sun, and to clean rooms while uninhabited; which is simply ignoring the first elementary notion of sanitary things, and laying the ground ready for all kinds of diseases.—3. That the window, and one window, is considered enough to air a room. Have you never observed that any room without a fire-place is always close? And, if you have a fire-place, would you cram it up not only with a chimney-board, but perhaps with a great wisp of brown paper, in the throat of the chimney—to prevent the soot from coming down, you say? If your chimney is foul, sweep it; but don't expect that you can ever air a room with only one aperture; don't suppose that to shut up a room is the way to keep it clean. It is the best way to foul the room and all that is in it. Don't imagine that if you, who are in charge, don't look to all these things yourself, those under you will be more careful than you are. It appears as if the part of a mistress now is to complain of her servants, and to accept their excuses—not to show them how there need be neither complaints made nor excuses.

Head in charge must see to House Hygiene, not do it herself.

But again, to look to all these things yourself, does not mean to do them yourself. "I always open the windows," the head in charge often says. If you do it, it is by so much the better, certainly, than if it were not done at all. But can you not insure that it is done when not done by yourself? Can you insure that it is not undone when your back is turned? This is what being "in charge" means. And a very important meaning it is, too. The former only implies that just what you can do with your own hands is done. The latter, that what ought to be done is always done.

Does God think of these things so seriously?

And now, you think these things trifles, or at least exaggerated.

But what you "think" or what I "think," matters little. Let us see what God thinks of them. God always justifies His ways. While we are "thinking," He has been teaching. I have known cases of hospital pyæmia quite as severe in handsome private houses as in any of the worst hospitals, and from the same cause, viz., foul air. Yet nobody learnt the lesson. Nobody learnt *anything* at all from it. They went on *thinking* —thinking that the sufferer had scratched his thumb, or that it was singular that "all the servants" had "whitlows," or that something was "much about this year; there is always sickness in our house." This is a favourite mode of thought—leading *not* to inquire what is the uniform cause of these general "whitlows," but to stifle all inquiry. In what sense is "sickness" being "always there," a justification of its being "there" at all?

14   What was the cause of hospital pyæmia being in that large private house? It was that the sewer air from an ill-placed sink was carefully conducted into all the rooms by sedulously opening all the doors, and closing all the passage windows. It was that the slops were emptied into the foot pans;—it was that the utensils were never properly rinsed;—it was that the chamber crockery was rinsed with dirty water;—it was that the beds were never properly shaken, aired, picked to pieces, or changed. It was that the carpets and curtains were always musty;—it was that the furniture was always dusty;—it was that the papered walls were saturated with dirt;—it was that the floors were never cleaned;—it was that the uninhabited rooms were never sunned, or cleaned, or aired;—it was that the cupboards were always reservoirs of foul air;—it was that the windows were always tight shut up at night;—it was that no window was ever systematically opened, even in the day, or that the right window was not opened. A person gasping for air might open a window for himself. But the servants were not taught to open the windows, to shut the doors; or they opened the windows upon a dank well between high walls, not upon the airier court; or they opened the room doors into the unaired halls and passages, by way of airing the rooms. Now all this is not fancy, but fact. In that handsome house there have been in one summer three cases of hospital pyæmia, one of phlebitis, two of consumptive cough: all the *immediate* products of foul air. When, in temperate climates, a house is more unhealthy in summer than in winter, it is a certain sign of something wrong. Yet nobody learns

How does He carry out His laws?

How does He teach His laws?

26 Health of Houses

the lesson. Yes, God always justifies His ways. He is teaching while you are not learning. This poor body loses his finger, that one loses his life. And all from the most easily preventible causes.

15   God lays down certain physical laws. Upon His carrying out such laws depends our responsibility (that much abused word), for how could we have any responsibility for actions, the results of which we could not foresee—which would be the case if the carrying out of His laws were not certain. Yet we seem to be continually expecting that He will work a miracle— *i.e.* break His own laws expressly to relieve us of responsibility.

16   "With God's Blessing he will recover," is a common form of parlance. But "with God's blessing" also, it is, if he does *not* recover; and "with God's blessing" that he fell ill; and "with God's blessing" that he dies, if he does die. In other words, *all* these things happen by God's laws, which *are* His blessings, that is, which are all to contribute to teach us the way to our best happiness. Cholera is just as much His "blessing" as the exemption from it. It is to teach us how to obey His laws, which are at once our means and our inducements to advance towards perfection. "With God's blessing he will recover," is a common form of speech with people who, all the while, are neglecting the means on which God has made health or recovery to depend.

Servants' rooms.

17   I must say a word about servants' bed-rooms. From the way they are built, but oftener from the way they are kept, and from no intelligent inspection whatever being exercised over them, they are almost invariably dens of foul air, and the "servants' health" suffers in an "unaccountable" (?) way, even in the country. For I am by no means speaking only of London houses, where too often servants are put to live under the ground and over the roof. But in a country " *mansion*," which was really a "mansion." (not after the fashion of advertisements), I have known three maids who slept in the same room ill of scarlet fever. "How catching it is!" was of course the remark. One look at the room, one smell of the room, was quite enough. It was no longer "unaccountable." The room was not a small one; it was up stairs, and it had two large windows—but nearly every one of the neglects enumerated above was there.

Physical degeneration in families. Its causes.

18   The houses of the grandmothers and great grandmothers of this generation, at least the country houses, with front door and back

door always standing open, winter and summer, and a thorough draught always blowing through—with all the scrubbing, and cleaning, and polishing, and scouring which used to go on, the grandmothers, and still more the great grandmothers, always out of doors and never with a bonnet on except to go to church, these things, when contrasted with our present "civilized" habits, entirely account for the fact so often seen of a great grandmother, who was a tower of physical vigour descending into a grandmother perhaps a little less vigorous but still sound as a bell and healthy to the core, into a mother languid and confined to her carriage and house, and lastly into a daughter sickly and confined to her bed. For, remember, even with a general decrease of mortality you may often find a race thus degenerating and still oftener a family. You may see poor little feeble washed-out rags, children of a noble stock, suffering morally and physically, throughout their useless, degenerate lives, and yet people who are going to marry and to bring more such into the world, will consult nothing but their own convenience as to where they are to live, or how they are to live.

19   That consumption is induced by the foul air of houses, *i.e.,* by air fouled by human bodies, more than by all other causes put together, is now certain. It is often alleged, even by physicians, as throwing doubt upon this fact, that "young ladies," who do not, it is supposed, live in a "vitiated atmosphere," yet die of consumption. But do these people know the up-stair habits of this class?—I do, or did. And of all classes there are two, viz., "young ladies," and soldiers, who are the most exposed to the influences which produce consumption. Both sleep, and partly live, in foul air. How many a time a young lady, advised to open her window and her curtains at night, says that "it would spoil her complexion." From this close, foul air both "young ladies" and soldiers go out at night in all weathers,—the one to "parties," the other to sentry duty; both enter into more foul air,—the one in crowded ball-rooms, the other in guard-rooms; both go home in damp night air after the skin and lungs have been oppressed in their functions by over crowding and want of ventilation, and both suffer from chest diseases, especially from consumption.

Consumption produced by foul air.

Both in soldiers and "young ladies."

20   Insufficient and unwholesome food is an auxiliary in some people to the work of consumption. For the "fashion" of not eating is still

28 Health of Houses

in vogue among "young ladies," and they make up for it, not unfrequently, in their own rooms, by tea and pound cake.

21 The object of spoiling her digestion is still further forwarded by many a young lady by the practice of taking continual and powerful aperients—still "to improve her complexion;" or, if the process of exhaustion is far advanced, by taking eau-de-Cologne, sal-volatile, or ether. It is little known how far this practice prevails.

22 Could we devise a course more likely first to ruin the general health and sow the seeds, and then act as a forcing-house to consumption?

Is consumption hereditary and inevitable?

23 Again, people often point to the frequency of consumption in some families to prove its "hereditary nature." Therefore it is inevitable. It is, indeed, extremely likely that if one or two deaths occur from consumption in a family there will be many more. For the whole family has been so mismanaged, that it is very unlikely that it should *not* attack other members in succession, just as children's epidemics do. But because seventeen persons, who eat poisoned sugar-plums at Bradford, several out of the same family, all die, is it a reason for supposing their poisoning "hereditary," "contagious," or the result of a "family predisposition?"

24 Again, some people say, we admit that two and a half times the number die of consumption in the army as die in civil life. But it is a mistake to suppose the cause of consumption in the army to be foul air, *for* the disease is "hereditary" in civil life.

25 *Therefore* Army surgeons select consumptive men for service, and "pass" two and a half times the number of recruits into the Army "predisposed" to consumption that exist in the civil population generally, and who would be rejected in the civil assurance offices? Is this the *Q.E.D.?*

26 Once more; it is indeed to be feared that weakness of digestion, or bad health *is* becoming "hereditary" in women of the upper classes, which also "predisposes" to consumption, and which, more than anything else, tends to the degeneracy of a family or race. Weakness of digestion depends upon habits; primarily and directly upon want of fresh air; secondarily and indirectly upon idleness or unhealthy excitement, unwholesome food, abuse of stimulants and aperients, and other exhausting habits.

Increase of births and of deaths in unhealthy districts.

27 Neglect of sanitary precautions is now generally admitted to be

a cause of disease in individuals and communities; but it is not so much known as it ought to be that the same neglect when continued in families tends to degrade the stock, and finally to destroy it. It has been often stated that intermarriage is a fruitful source of family degradation; but is it considered that other habits descending from parents to offspring, such, for instance, as intemperance, breathing foul air, living in gloomy unhealthy localities and the like, also tend to degeneration? We have important indirect statistical proof of the operation of this law on comparing the proportion of births to the proportion of deaths in "registration" districts, under opposite sanitary conditions.

28 In healthy "registration" districts, the mortality is low and the annual proportion of births is also low, but in unhealthy districts the mortality rises, while at the same time the proportion of births increases, showing that in such districts the circuit of life is shortened.

29 The table of deaths and births in the 10 years, 1841-50, in six of the most healthy and in six of the least healthy districts in England, given below, illustrates the law.*

*Table of Deaths and Births in Healthy and Unhealthy Districts.		
Districts.	To 1000 persons living.	
	Deaths.	Births.
Rothbury (Northumberland)	15	24
Glendale Do.	15	31
Eastbourne (Sussex)	15	30
Holsworthy (Devon)	16	30
Battle (Sussex)	16	33
Reigate (Surrey)	16	31
Mean	$15\frac{1}{2}$	30
Liverpool (Lancashire)	36	40
Manchester Do.	33	37
St. Saviour's, Southwark	33	37
Hull (York)	31	30
St. George's, Southwark	30	35
Leeds (York)	30	36
Mean	32	36

30 Health of Houses

30   It would appear from this table that a double mortality is attended by an increase of births to the extent of 20 per cent.

31   The Registrar-General showed in his fifth annual report (1843) that a similar law prevails for the healthy and unhealthy districts of the Metropolis. In the unhealthiest sub-districts, the deaths per 1,000 were 29. 9, and the births per 1,000 were 35. 2, while in the healthiest sub-districts the deaths per 1,000 were 18. and the births per 1,000 were 24. This increase of births among unhealthy populations has been long known to sanitary observers, and has been thought to point to another law, namely that of a constant endeavour to preserve the race or family, the existence of which has been endangered by man's neglect of the laws on which its existence depends.

32   Now as to these children ushered into existence in the midst of such excessive mortality?

33   Has not every one had the opportunity of comparing the full healthy development of a child born in these healthy country districts with the thin, ill fed, undeveloped or ill-developed frame of the child born in unhealthy towns? And is not the conclusion irresistible that the unhealthy town child belongs to a lower family type than the healthy country child? A process of physical degradation has been going on notwithstanding the increase of births, and of these two classes of children about a third of the country children die before they reach the age of five years, while of the town children a half die before that period, and a large proportion of those who survive their fifth year are puny sickly people whose early deaths go to swell the local mortality.

34   These are momentous facts, if people would only ponder them, and act on the lessons they are teaching.

Don't make your sick-room into a ventilating shaft for the whole house.

35   With regard to the health of houses where there is a sick person, it often happens that the sick room is made a ventilating shaft for the rest of the house. For while the house is kept as close, unaired, and dirty as usual, the window of the sick room is kept a little open always, and the door occasionally. Now, there are certain sacrifices which a house with one sick person in it does make to that sick person: it ties up its knocker; it lays straw before it in the street. Why can't it keep itself thoroughly clean and unusually well aired, in deference to the sick person?

Infection.

36   We must not forget what, in ordinary language, is called "Infec-

tion;"—a thing of which people are generally so afraid that they frequently follow the very practice in regard to it which they ought to avoid. Nothing used to be considered so infectious or contagious as small pox; and people, not very long ago, used to cover up patients with heavy bed clothes, while they kept up large fires and shut the windows. Small pox, of course, under this *régime*, was very "infectious." People are somewhat wiser now in their management of this disease. They have ventured to cover the patients lightly and to keep the windows open; and we hear much less of the "infection" of small pox than we used to do. But do people in our days act with more wisdom on the subject of "infection" in fevers—scarlet fever, measles, &c.—than their forefathers did with small pox? Does not the popular idea of "infection" involve that people should take greater care of themselves than of the patient? that, for instance, it is safer not to be too much with the patient, not to attend too much to his wants? Perhaps the best illustration of the utter absurdity of this view of duty in attending on "infectious" diseases is afforded by what was very recently the practice, if it is not so even now, in some of the European lazarets—in which the plague-patient used to be condemned to the horrors of filth, overcrowding, and want of ventilation, while the medical attendant was ordered to examine the patient's tongue through an opera-glass and to toss him a lancet to open his abscesses with!

37   True nursing ignores infection, except to prevent it. Cleanliness and fresh air from open windows, with unremitting attention to the patient, are the only defence a true nurse either asks or needs.

38   Wise and humane management of the patient is the best safeguard against infection.

39   Is it not living in a continual mistake to look upon diseases, as we do now, as separate entities, which *must* exist, like cats and dogs? instead of looking upon them as conditions, like a dirty and a clean condition, and just as much under our own control; or rather as the reactions of a kindly nature, against the conditions in which we have placed ourselves.

Diseases are not individuals arranged in classes, like cats and dogs, but conditions growing out of one another.

40   I was brought up, both by scientific men and ignorant women, distinctly to believe that small pox, for instance, was a thing of which there was once a first specimen in the world, which went on propagating itself, in a perpetual chain of descent, just as much as that

there was a first dog, (or a first pair of dogs), and that small pox would not begin itself any more than a new dog would begin without there having been a parent dog.

41   Since then I have seen with my eyes and smelt with my nose small pox growing up in first specimens, either in close rooms or in overcrowded wards, where it could not by any possibility have been "caught," but must have begun.

42   Nay, more, I have seen diseases begin, grow up, and pass into one another. Now, dogs do not pass into cats.

43   I have seen, for instance, with a little overcrowding, continued fever grow up; and with a little more, typhoid fever; and with a little more, typhus, and all in the same ward or hut.

44   Would it not be far better, truer, and more practical if we looked upon disease in this light?

45   For diseases, as all experience shows, are adjectives, not noun substantives.

Why must children have measles, &c.?

46   There are not a few popular opinions, in regard to which it is useful at times to ask a question or two. For example, it is commonly thought that children must have what are commonly called "children's epidemics," "current contagions," &c.; in other words, that they are born to have measles, hooping-cough, perhaps even scarlet fever, just as they are born to cut their teeth, if they live.

47   Now, do tell us, why must a child have measles?

48   Oh, because, you say, we cannot keep it from infection—other children have measles—and it must take them—and it is safer that it should.

49   But why must other children have measles? And if they have, why must yours have them too?

50   If you believed in and observed the laws for preserving the health of houses which inculcate cleanliness, ventilation, white-washing, and other means, and which, by the way, *are laws,* as implicitly as you believe in the popular opinion, for it is nothing more than an opinion, that your child must have children's epidemics, don't you think that, upon the whole, your child would be more likely to escape altogether?

III. PETTY MANAGEMENT.

1   All the results of good nursing, as detailed in these notes, may be spoiled or utterly negatived by one defect, viz.: in petty management, or, in other words, by not knowing how to manage, that what you do when you are there shall be done when you are not there. The most devoted friend or nurse cannot be always *there*. Nor is it desirable that she should. And she may give up her health, all her other duties, and yet, for want of a little management, be not one-half so efficient as another who is not one-half so devoted, but who has this art of multiplying herself—that is to say, the patient of the first will not really be so well cared for as the patient of the second.

2   It is as impossible in a book to teach a person in charge of sick how to *manage,* as it is to teach her how to nurse. Circumstances must vary with each different case. But it *is* possible to press upon her to think for herself. Now, what does happen during my absence? I am obliged to be away on Tuesday. But fresh air, or punctuality, is not less important to my patient on Tuesday than it was on Monday. Or: At 10 p.m. I am never with my patient; but quiet is of no less consequence to him at 10 than it was at 5 minutes to 10.

3   Curious as it may seem, this very obvious consideration occurs comparatively to few, or, if it does occur, it is only to cause the devoted friend or nurse to be absent fewer hours or fewer minutes from her patient—not to arrange so as that no minute and no hour shall be for her patient without the essentials of her nursing.

Petty management.

4 A very few instances will be sufficient, not as precepts, but as illustrations.

Illustrations of the want of it.

5 A strange washerwoman, coming late at night for the "things," will burst in by mistake to the patient's sick-room, after he has fallen into his first doze, giving him a shock, the effects of which are irremediable, though he himself laughs at the cause, and probably never even mentions it. The nurse who is, and is quite right to be, at her supper, has not provided that the washerwoman shall not lose her way and go into the wrong room.

Strangers coming into the sick room.

6 The patient's room may always have the window open. But the passage outside the patient's room, though provided with several large windows, may never have one open. Because it is not understood that the charge of the sick-room extends to the charge of the passage. And thus, as often happens, the nurse makes it her business to turn the patient's room into a ventilating shaft for the foul air of the whole house.

Sick room airing the whole house.

7 An uninhabited room, a newly painted room, an uncleaned closet or cupboard, may often become a reservoir of foul air for the whole house, because the person in charge never thinks of arranging that these places shall be always aired, always cleaned; she merely opens the window herself "when she goes in."

Uninhabited room fouling the whole house.

8 That excellent paper, the *Builder*, mentions the lingering of the smell of paint for a month about a house as a proof of want of ventilation. Certainly—and, where there are ample windows to open, and these are never opened to get rid of the smell of paint, it is a proof of want of management in using the means of ventilation. Of course the smell will then remain for months. Why should it go?

Lingering smell of paint a want of care.

9 An agitating letter or message may be delivered, or an important letter or message *not* delivered; a visitor whom it was of consequence to see, may be refused, or one whom it was of still more consequence *not* to see may be admitted—because the person in charge has never asked herself this question. What is done when I am not there?

Delivery and non-delivery of letters and messages.

10 Why should you let your patient ever be surprised, except by thieves? I do not know. In England, people do not come down the chimney, or through the window, unless they are thieves. They come in by the door, and somebody must open the door to them. The "somebody" charged with opening the door is one of two, three, or at most

Why let your patient ever be surprised?

four persons. Why cannot these, at most, four persons be put in charge as to what is to be done when there is a ring at the door bell?

11 The sentry at a post is changed much oftener than any servant at a private house or institution can possibly be. But what should we think of such an excuse as this: that the enemy had entered such a post because A and not B had been on guard? Yet such an excuse is constantly heard in the private house or institution and accepted: viz., that such a person had been "let in" or *not* "let in," and such a parcel had been wrongly delivered or lost because A and not B had opened the door!

12 At all events, one may safely say, a nurse cannot be with the patient, open the door, eat her meals, take a message, all at one and the same time. Nevertheless the person in charge never seems to look the impossibility in the face.

13 Add to this that the *attempting* this impossibility does more to increase the poor patient's hurry and nervousness than anything else.

14 It is never thought that the patient remembers these things if you do not. He has not only to think whether the visit or letter may arrive, but whether you will be in the way at the particular day and hour when it may arrive. So that your *partial* measures for "being in the way" yourself, only increase the necessity for his thought. Whereas, if you could but arrange that the thing should always be done whether you are there or not, he need never think at all about it.

Partial measures such as "being always in the way" yourself, increase instead of saving the patient's anxiety. Because they must be only partial.

15 For the above reasons, whatever a patient can do for himself, it is better, *i.e.* less anxiety, for him to do for himself, unless the person in charge has the spirit of management.

16 It is evidently much less exertion for a patient to answer a letter for himself by return of post, than to have four conversations, wait five days, have six anxieties before it is off his mind, before the person who is to answer it has done so.

17 Apprehension, uncertainty, waiting, expectation, fear of surprise, do a patient more harm than any exertion. Remember, he is face to face with his enemy all the time, internally wrestling with him, having long imaginary conversations with him. You are thinking of something else. "Rid him of his adversary quickly," is a first rule with the sick.

18 There are many physical operations where *cœteris paribus* the

36   Petty Management

danger is in a direct ratio to the time the operation lasts; and *cæteris paribus* the operator's success will be in direct ratio to his quickness. Now there are many mental operations where exactly the same rule holds good with the sick; *cæteris paribus* their capability of bearing such operations depends directly on the quickness, *without hurry*, with which they can be got through.

19   For the same reasons, always tell a patient and tell him beforehand when you are going out and when you will be back, whether it is for a day, an hour, or ten minutes. You fancy perhaps that it is better for him if he does not find out your going at all, better for him if you do not make yourself "of too much importance" to him; or else you cannot bear to give him the pain or the anxiety of the temporary separation.

20   No such thing. You *ought* to go, we will suppose. Health or duty requires it. Then say so to the patient openly. If you go without his knowing it, and he finds it out, he never will feel secure again that the things which depend upon you will be done when you are away, and in nine cases out of ten he will be right. If you go out without telling him when you will be back, he can take no measures nor precautions as to the things which concern you both, or which you do for him.

<small>What is the cause of half the accidents which happen?</small>

21   If you look into the reports of trials or accidents, and especially of suicides, or into the medical history of fatal cases, it is almost incredible how often the whole thing turns upon something which has happened because "he," or still oftener "she," "was not there." But it is still more incredible how often, how almost always this is accepted as a sufficient reason, a justification; why, the very fact of the thing having happened is the proof of its not being a justification. The person in charge was quite right not to be "*there*" he was called away for quite sufficient reason, or he was away for a daily recurring and unavoidable cause: yet no provision was made to supply his absence. The fault was not in his "being away," but in there being no management to supplement his "being away." When the sun is under a total eclipse, or during his nightly absence, we light candles. But it would seem as if it did not occur to us that we must also supplement the person in charge of sick or of children, whether under an occasional eclipse or during a regular absence.

22   In institutions where many lives would be lost, and the effect of

such want of management would be terrible and patent, there is less of it than in the private house.

23 So true is this, that I could mention two cases of women of very high position, both of whom died in the same way of the consequences of a surgical operation. And in both cases I was told by the highest authority that the fatal result would not have happened in a London hospital.

Petty management better understood in institutions than in private houses.

24 But, as far as regards the art of petty management in hospitals, all the military hospitals I know must be excluded. Upon my own experience I stand, and I solemnly declare that I have seen or known of fatal accidents, such as suicides in *delirium tremens*,* bleedings to death, dying patients dragged out of bed by drunken Medical Staff Corps men, and many other things less patent and striking, which would not have happened in London civil hospitals nursed by women. The medical officers should be absolved from all blame in these accidents. How can a medical officer mount guard all day and all night over a patient (say) in *delirium tremens ?* The fault lies in there being no organized system of attendance. Were a trustworthy *man* in charge of each ward, or set of wards, not as office clerk, but as head nurse (and head nurse the best hospital serjeant, or ward master, is not now and cannot be, from default of the proper regulations), the thing would not, in all probability, have happened. But were a trustworthy *woman* in charge of the ward, or set of wards, the thing would not, in all certainty, have happened. In other words, it does not happen where a trustworthy woman is really in charge. And, in these remarks, I by no means refer only to exceptional times of great emergency in war hospitals, but also, and quite as much, to the ordinary run of military hospitals at home, in time of peace; or to a time in war when our army was actually more healthy than at home in peace, and the pressure on our hospitals consequently much less.

What institutions are the exception ?

25 It is often said that, in regimental hospitals, patients ought to

Nursing in Regimental Hospitals.

(24) * Note.—The simple precaution of removing cords by which a patient can hang himself, razors by which he can cut his throat, out of his way, when inclined to do such things, is much neglected especially in private nursing. Many inquests upon suicides shew this, and the friends are invariably absolved by the verdict. In a Military Hospital, an officer of rank cut his own throat, in delirium tremens, with a razor which no one ever thought of removing. Who among us has not some melancholy experience similar, although not identical ?

"nurse each other," because the number of sick altogether being, say, but thirty, and out of these one only perhaps being seriously ill, and the other twenty-nine having little the matter with them, and nothing to do, they should be set to nurse the one; also, that soldiers are so trained to obey, that they will be the most obedient, and therefore the best of nurses, add to which they are always kind to their comrades.

26 Now, have those who say this, considered that, in order to obey, you must know *how* to obey, and that these soldiers certainly do not know how to obey in nursing. I have seen these "kind" fellows (and how kind they are no one knows so well as myself) move a comrade so that, in one case at least, the man died in the act. I have seen the comrades' "kindness" produce abundance of spirits, to be drunk in secret. Let no one understand by this that female nurses ought to, or could be introduced in regimental hospitals. It would be most undesirable, even were it not impossible. But the head nurseship of a hospital serjeant is the more essential, the more inexperienced the "orderlies." Undoubtedly, a London hospital "sister" does sometimes set relays of patients to watch a critical case; but, undoubtedly also, always under her own superintendence; and she is called to whenever there is something to be done, and she knows how to do it. The patients are not left to do it of their own unassisted genius, however "kind" and willing they may be.

<small>Question for persons "in charge."</small>

27 In both, the institution and the private house, let whoever is in charge keep this simple question in her head (*not,* how can I always do this right thing myself? but), how can I provide for this right thing to be always done?

28 Then, when anything wrong has actually happened in consequence of her absence, which absence we will suppose to have been quite right, let her question still be (*not,* how can I provide against any of such absences? which is neither possible nor desirable, but), how can I provide against any thing wrong arising out of my absence?

29 Many people seem to think that the world stands still while they are away, or at dinner, or ill. If the sick have an accident during that time, is it their fault, not yours? I once heard an official justly told, "Patients, Sir, will not stop dying, while we are in church."

30 It is the invariable sign of a bad nurse and manager when her excuse that such a person was neglected or such a thing was left undone, is, that she was "out of the way." What does that signify?

The thing that signifies is that the neglect should not happen.

31   How few men, or even women, understand, either in great or in little things, what it is the being "in charge"—I mean, know how to carry out a "charge." From the most colossal calamities, down to the most trifling accidents, results are often traced (or rather *not* traced) to such want of some one "in charge" or of his knowing how to be "in charge." A short time ago the bursting of a funnel-casing on board the finest and strongest ship that ever was built, on her trial trip, destroyed several lives, and put several hundreds in jeopardy—not from any undetected flaw in her new and untried works—but from a tap being closed which ought not to have been closed—from what every child knows would make its mother's tea-kettle burst. And this simply because no one seemed to know what it is to be "in charge," or *who* was in charge. Nay more, the jury at the inquest actually altogether ignored the same, and apparently considered the tap "in charge," for they gave as a verdict "accidental death."

What it is to be "in charge."

32   This is the meaning of the word, on a large scale. On a much smaller scale, it happened, a short time ago, that an insane person burnt herself slowly and intentionally to death, while in her doctor's charge, and almost in his nurse's presence. Yet neither was considered "at all to blame." The very fact of the accident happening proves its own case. There is nothing more to be said. Either they did not know their business, or they did not know how to perform it.

33   To be "in charge" is certainly not only to carry out the proper measures yourself but to see that every one else does so too; to see that no one either wilfully or ignorantly thwarts or prevents such measures. It is neither to do everything yourself, nor to appoint a number of people to each duty, but to ensure that each does that duty to which he is appointed. This is the meaning which must be attached to the word by (above all) those "in charge" of sick, whether of numbers or of individuals, (and indeed I think it is with individual sick that it is least understood. One sick person is often waited on by four with less precision, and is really less cared for than ten who are waited on by one; or at least than forty who are waited on by four; and all for want of this one person "in charge.")

34   It is often said that there are few good servants now: I say there are few good mistresses now. As the jury seems to have thought the

40 Petty Management

tap was in charge of the ship's safety, so mistresses now seem to think the house is in charge of itself. They neither know how to give orders, nor how to teach servants to obey orders— *i.e.* to obey intelligently, which is the real meaning of all discipline.

35   Again, people who are in charge often seem to have a pride in feeling that they will be "missed," that no one can understand or carry on their arrangements, their system, books, accounts, &c., but themselves. It seems to me that the pride is rather in carrying on a system, in keeping stores, closets, books, accounts, &c., so that anybody can understand and carry them on—so that, in case of absence or illness, one can deliver everything up to others and know that all will go on as usual, and one shall never be missed.

Why hired nurses give trouble.

36   It is often complained, that professional nurses, brought into private families, in case of sickness, make themselves intolerable by "ordering about" the other servants, under plea of not neglecting the patient. Both things are true; the patient is often neglected, and the servants are often unfairly "put upon." But the fault is generally in the want of management of the head in charge. It is surely for her to arrange both that the nurse's place is, when necessary, supplemented, and that the patient is never neglected—things with a little management quite compatible, and, indeed, only attainable together. It is certainly not for the nurse to "order about" the servants.

37   In being asked to recommend a sick-nurse, what is it one is asked for? To send a nurse to save the patient's friends from "sitting up;" to save the servant from "running up and down stairs;" not to ensure the patient being better nursed. Physicians of large practice have assured me that their experience was the same.

Nurses not expected to "nurse"— reason why there are few good ones.

38   Surely here is the root of the whole matter. People's object in having a nurse is *not* that she should "nurse,"—they do not know what "nursing" is,—they want a drudge. The "running up and down stairs," the "sitting up," are indeed unmercifully exacted of the poor individual called a nurse. I should call her a *lift*.

39   No wonder there is little or no good nursing in private families.

40   A nurse should do nothing but nurse. If you want a charwoman, have one. Nursing is a specialty. Army doctors used to be asked to sit in judgment on stores and accounts, and to overlook washing bills. Happily for the sick, army doctors are now set free for their professional duties. Are the duties of the nurse, though subordinate,

less important?

41 *How to be ill* is certainly an essential complement of *how to nurse*. One part of the subject is not complete without the other. But on the whole the first duty is generally better performed than the second.

42 There is one point, however, on the other side, in which, according to the experience of all people and institutions who send out nurses, the sick, or perhaps oftener the friends of the sick, lamentably fail. And this is in expecting nurses to "sit up" night after night without any proper provision for ensuring to them quiet and regular sleep during the day. In sending out a nurse a precise bargain must always be made for her sleep.

IV. NOISE.

¹ Unnecessary noise, or noise that creates an expectation in the mind, is that which hurts a patient. It is rarely the loudness of the noise, the effect upon the organ of the ear itself, which appears to affect the sick. How well a patient will generally bear, *e.g.,* the putting up of a scaffolding close to the house, when he cannot bear the talking still less the whispering, especially if it be of a familiar voice, outside his door. Unnecessary noise.

² There are certain patients, no doubt, especially where there is slight concussion or other disturbance of the brain, who are affected by mere noise. But intermittent noise, or sudden and sharp noise, in these as in all other cases, affects far more than continuous noise—noise with jar far more than noise without. Of one thing you may be certain, that anything which wakes a patient suddenly out of his sleep will invariably put him into a state of greater excitement, do him more serious, aye, and lasting mischief, than any continuous noise, however loud.

³ Never to allow a patient to be waked, intentionally or accidentally, is a *sine qua non* of all good nursing. If he is roused out of his first sleep, he is almost certain to have no more sleep. It is a curious but quite intelligible fact that, if a patient is waked after a few hours' instead of a few minutes' sleep, he is much more likely to sleep again. Because pain, like irritability of brain, perpetuates and intensifies itself. If you have gained a respite of either in sleep you have gained Never let a patient be waked out of his first sleep.

44 Noise

more than the mere respite. Both the probability of recurrence and of the same intensity will be diminished, whereas both will be terribly increased by want of sleep. This is the reason why sleep is so all-important. This is the reason why a patient, waked in the early part of his sleep, loses, not only his sleep, but his power to sleep. A healthy person who allows himself to sleep during the day will lose his sleep at night. But it is exactly the reverse with the sick generally; the more they sleep the better will they be able to sleep.

4   A good nurse can apply hot bottles to the feet, or give the nourishment ordered, hour by hour, without disturbing, but rather composing the patient. I have seen one of the (would be) careful nurses neglect to warm the legs of a patient, invariably cold in the early morning, because "she did not like to disturb him." Such an excuse stamps a woman at once as incapable of her trust.

Noise which excites expectation.

5   I have often been surprised at the thoughtlessness, (resulting in cruelty, quite unintentional), of friend or of doctor who will hold a long conversation just in the room or passage adjoining to the room of the patient, who is either every moment expecting them to come in, or who has just seen them, and knows they are talking about him. If he is an amiable patient, he will try to occupy his attention elsewhere and not to listen—and this makes matters worse—for the strain upon his attention and the effort he makes are so great that it is well if he is not worse for hours after. *Whispered conversation in the room* If it is a whispered conversation in the same room, then it is absolutely cruel; for it is impossible that the patient's attention should not be involuntarily strained to hear. Walking on tip-toe, doing anything in the room very slowly, are injurious, for exactly the same reasons. A firm light quick step, a steady quick hand are the desiderata; not the slow, lingering, shuffling foot, the timid, uncertain touch. Slowness is not gentleness, though it is often mistaken for such; quickness, lightness, and gentleness are quite compatible. Again, if friends and doctors did but watch, as nurses can and should watch, the features sharpening, the eyes growing almost wild, of fever patients who are listening for the entrance from the corridor of the persons whose voices they are hearing there, these would never run the risk again of creating such expectation, or irritation of mind. Such unnecessary noise has undoubtedly induced or aggravated delirium in many cases. I have known such. In one ease death ensued. It is but fair to say that

this death was attributed to fright. It was the result of a long whispered conversation, within sight of the patient, about an impending operation; but any one who has known the more than stoicism, the cheerful coolness, with which the certainty of an operation will be accepted by any patient, capable of bearing an operation at all, if it is properly communicated to him, will hesitate to believe that it was mere fear which produced, as was averred, the fatal result in this instance. It was rather the uncertainty, the strained expectation as to what was to be decided upon.

6   I need hardly say that the other common course, namely, for a doctor or friend to leave the patient and communicate his opinion on the result of his visit to the friends just outside the patient's door, or inside the adjoining room, after the visit, but within hearing or knowledge of the patient is, if possible, worst of all. *(Or just outside the door.)*

7   Affectation, like whispering or walking on tiptoe, is peculiarly painful to the sick. An affectedly quiet voice, an affectedly sympathising voice, like an undertaker's at a funeral, sets all their nerves on edge. Advice, such as what I have been giving, does more harm than good, if it only makes people *affect* composure and quiet, when with the sick. Better almost make your natural noise. *(Affectation.)*

8   It is, I think, alarming, peculiarly at this time, when the female ink-bottles are perpetually impressing upon us "woman's" "particular worth and general missionariness," to see that the dress of woman is daily more and more unfitting them for any "mission," or usefulness at all. It is equally unfitted for all poetic and all domestic purposes. A man is now a more handy and far less objectionable being in a sick room than a woman. Compelled by her dress, every woman now either shuffles or waddles—only a man can cross the floor of a sick room without shaking it! What is become of woman's light step?—the firm, light, quick step we have been asked for? *(Noise of female dress.)*

9   Lord Melbourne said "I would rather have men about me when I am ill; I think it requires very strong health to put up with women." I am quite of his opinion.

10   Unnecessary noise, then, is the most cruel absence of care which can be inflicted either on sick or well. For, in all these remarks, the sick are only mentioned as suffering in a greater proportion than the well from precisely the same causes.

11   Unnecessary (although slight) noise injures a sick person much

more than necessary noise (of a much greater amount).

12 All doctrines about mysterious affinities and aversions will be found to resolve themselves very much, if not entirely, into presence or absence of care in these things.

Patient's repulsion to nurses who rustle.

13 A nurse who rustles (I am speaking of nurses professional and unprofessional) is the horror of a patient, though perhaps he does not know why.

14 The fidget of silk and of crinoline, the crackling of starched petticoats, the rattling of keys, the creaking of stays and of shoes, will do a patient more harm than all the medicines in the world will do him good.

15 The noiseless step of woman, the noiseless drapery of woman, are mere figures of speech in this day. Her skirts (and well if they do not throw down some piece of furniture) will at least brush against every article in the room as she moves.

Burning of the crinolines.

16 Fortunate it is if her skirts do not catch fire—and if the nurse does not give herself up a sacrifice together with her patient, to be burnt in her own petticoats. I wish the Registrar-General would tell us the exact number of deaths by burning occasioned by this absurd and hideous custom. But if people will be stupid, let them take measures to protect themselves from their own stupidity—measures which every chemist knows, such as putting alum into starch, which prevents starched articles of dress from blazing up.

Indecency of the crinolines.

17 I wish too that people who wear crinoline could see the indecency of their own dress as other people see it. A respectable elderly woman stooping forward, invested in crinoline, exposes quite as much of her own person to the patient lying in the room as any opera dancer does on the stage. But no one will ever tell her this unpleasant truth.

Patients obliged to defend themselves against their nurses.

18 Again, one nurse cannot open the door without making everything rattle. Or she opens the door unnecessarily often, for want of remembering all the articles that might be brought in at once.

19 I have seen an expression of real terror pass across a patient's face, whenever a nurse came into the room who stumbled over the fire irons, &c.

20 I have seen patients, scarcely able to crawl, get out of bed before such a nurse came in and put out of her way everything she could throw down,—shut the window, sure that she would leave the door

open—hide everything they were likely to want, (not because they had no right to have it, but because she would inadvertently put it out of their reach).

21   A good nurse will always make sure that no door or window in her patient's room shall rattle or creak; that no blind or curtain shall, by any change of wind through the open window, be made to flap—especially will she be careful of all this before she leaves her patients for the night. If you wait till your patients tell you, or remind you of these things, where is the use of their having a nurse? There are more shy than exacting patients, in all classes; and many a patient passes a bad night, time after time, rather than remind his nurse every night of all the things she has forgotten.

22   If there are blinds to your windows always take care to have them well up, when they are not being used. A little piece slipping down, and flapping with every draught, will distract a patient.

23   All hurry or bustle is peculiarly painful to the sick. And when a patient has compulsory occupations to engage him, intead of having simply to amuse himself, it becomes doubly injurious. The friend who remains standing and fidgeting about while a patient is talking business to him, or the friend who sits and proses, the one from an idea of not letting the patient talk, the other from an idea of amusing him,—each is equally inconsiderate. Always sit down when a sick person is talking business to you, show no signs of hurry, give complete attention and full consideration if your advice is wanted, and go away the moment the subject is ended. *Hurry peculiarly hurtful to sick.*

24   Always sit within the patient's view, so that when you speak to him he has not painfully to turn his head round in order to look at you. Everybody involuntarily looks at the person speaking. If you make this act a wearisome one on the part of the patient you are doing him harm. So also if by continuing to stand you make him continuously raise his eyes to see you. Be as motionless as possible, and never gesticulate in speaking to the sick. *How to visit the sick and not hurt them.*

25   Never make a patient repeat a message or request, especially if it be some time after. Occupied patients are often accused of doing too much of their own business. They are instinctively right. How often you hear the person, charged with the request of giving the message or writing the letter, say half an hour afterwards to the patient, "Did you appoint 12 o'clock?" or "What did you say was the

48 Noise

address?" or ask perhaps some much more agitating question—thus causing the patient the effort of memory, or worse still, of decision, all over again. It is really less exertion to him to write his letters himself. This is the almost universal experience of occupied invalids.

26 This brings us to another caution. Never speak to an invalid from behind, nor from the door, nor from any distance from him, nor when he is doing anything.

27 The official politeness of servants in these things is so grateful to invalids, that many prefer, without knowing why, having none but servants about them.

These things not fancy.

28 These things are not fancy. If we consider that, with sick as with well, every thought decomposes some nervous matter,—that decomposition as well as recomposition of nervous matter is always going on, and more quickly with the sick than with the well,—that do obtrude abruptly another thought upon the brain while it is in the act of destroying nervous matter by thinking, is calling upon it to make a new exertion,—if we consider these things, which are facts, not fancies, we shall remember that we are doing positive injury by interrupting, by "startling a fanciful" person, as it is called. Alas! it is no fancy.

Interruption damaging to sick.

29 If the invalid is forced, by his avocations, to continue occupations requiring much thinking, the injury is doubly great. In feeding a patient suffering under delirium or stupor you may suffocate him, by giving him his food suddenly; but if you rub his lips gently with a spoon, and thus attract his attention, he will swallow the food unconsciously, but with perfect safety. Thus it is with the brain. If you offer it a thought, especially one requiring a decision, abruptly, you do it a real not fanciful injury. Never speak to a sick person suddenly; but, at the same time, do not keep his expectation on the tip-toe.

And to well.

30 This rule, indeed, applies to the well quite as much as to the sick. I have never known persons who exposed themselves for years to constant interruption who did not muddle away their intellects by it at last. The process with them may be accomplished without pain. With the sick, pain gives warning of the injury.

Keeping a patient standing.

31 Do not meet or overtake a patient who is moving about in order to speak to him, or to give him any message or letter. You might just as well give him a box on the ear. I have seen a patient fall flat on the ground who was standing when his nurse came into the room.

This was an accident which might have happened to the most careful nurse. But the other is done with intention. A patient in such a state is not going to the East Indies. If you would wait ten seconds, or walk ten yards further, any promenade he could make would be over. You do not know the effort it is to a patient to remain standing for even a quarter of a minute to listen to you. If I had not seen the thing done by the kindest nurses and friends, I should have thought this caution quite superfluous.

32   It is absolutely essential then that a nurse should lay this down as a positive rule to herself, never to speak to any patient who is standing or moving, as long as she exercises so little observation as not to know when a patient cannot bear it. Many of the accidents which happen from feeble patients tumbling down stairs, fainting after getting up, &c., happen solely from the nurse popping out of a door to speak to the patient just at that moment; or from his fearing that she will do so. And that if the patient were even left to himself, till he can sit down, such accidents would much seldomer occur. If the nurse accompanies the patient let her not call upon him to speak. It is incredible that nurses cannot picture to themselves the strain upon the heart, the lungs, and the brain which the act of moving is to any feeble patient. *[Never speak to a patient in the act of moving.]*

33   Patients are often accused of being able to "do much more when nobody is by." It is quite true that they can. Unless nurses can be brought to attend to considerations of the kind of which we have given here but a few specimens, a very weak patient finds it really much less exertion to do things for himself than to ask for them. And he will, in order to do them, (very innocently and from instinct) calculate the time his nurse is likely to be absent, from a fear of her "coming in upon" him or speaking to him, just at the moment when he finds it quite as much as he can do to crawl from his bed to his chair, or from one room to another, or down stairs, or out of doors for a few minutes. Some extra call made upon his attention at that moment will quite upset him. In these cases you may be sure that a patient in the state we have described does not make such exertions more than once or twice a-day, and probably much about the same hour every day. And it is hard, indeed, if nurse and friends cannot calculate so as to let him make them undisturbed. Remember, that many patients can walk who cannot stand or even sit up. Standing is, *[Patients dread surprise.]*

of all positions, the most trying to a weak patient.

34 Everything you do in a patient's room, after he is "put up" for the night, increases tenfold the risk of his having a bad night. But, if you rouse him up after he has fallen asleep, you do not risk, you secure him a bad night.

35 One hint I would give to all who attend or visit the sick, to all who have to pronounce an opinion upon sickness or its progress. Come back and look at your patient *after* he has had an hour's animated conversation with you. It is the best test of his real state we know. But never pronounce upon him from merely seeing what he does, or how he looks, during such a conversation. Learn also carefully and exactly, if you can, how he passed the night after it.

Effects of over-exertion on sick.

36 People rarely, if ever, faint while making an exertion. It is after it is over. Indeed, almost every effect of over-exertion appears after, not during such exertion. It is the highest folly to judge of the sick, as is so often done, when you see them merely during a period of excitement. People have very often died of that which, it has been proclaimed at the time, has "done them no harm."

Careless observation of the results of careless visits.

37 As an old experienced nurse, I do most earnestly deprecate all such careless words. I have known patients delirious all night, after seeing a visitor who called them "better," thought they "only wanted a little amusement," and who came again, saying, "I hope you were not the worse for my visit," neither waiting for an answer, nor even looking at the case. No real patient will ever say, "Yes, but I was a great deal the worse."

38 It is not, however, either death or delirium of which, in these cases, there is most danger to the patient. Unperceived consequences are far more likely to ensue. *You* will have impunity—the poor patient will *not.* That is, the patient will suffer, although neither he nor the inflictor of the injury will attribute it to its real cause. It will not be directly traceable, except by a very careful observant nurse. The patient will often not even mention what has done him most harm.

Don't lean upon the sick-bed.

39 Remember never to lean against, sit upon, or unnecessarily shake, or even touch the bed in which a patient lies. This is invariably a painful annoyance. If you shake the chair on which he sits, he has a point by which to steady himself, in his feet. But on a bed or sofa, he is entirely at your mercy, and he feels every jar you give him all

through him.

40 In all that we have said, both here and elsewhere, let it be distinctly understood that we are not speaking of hypochondriacs. To distinguish between real and fancied disease forms an important branch of education of a nurse. To manage fancy patients forms an important branch of her duties. But the nursing which real and that which fancied patients require is of different, or rather of opposite, character. And the latter will not be spoken of here. Indeed, many of the symptoms which are here mentioned are those which distinguish real from fancied disease. *Difference between real and fancy patients.*

41 It is true that hypochondriacs very often do that behind a nurse's back which they would not do before her face. Many such I have had as patients who scarcely ate anything at their regular meals; but if you concealed food for them in a drawer, they would take it at night or in secret. But this is from quite a different motive. They do it from the wish to conceal. Whereas the real patient will often boast to his nurse or doctor, if these do not shake their heads at him, of how much he has done, or eaten, or walked. To return to real disease.

42 Conciseness and decision are, above all things, necessary with the sick. Let your thought expressed to them be concisely and decidedly expressed. What doubt and hesitation there may be in your own mind must never be communicated to theirs, not even (I would rather say especially not) in little things. Let your doubt be to yourself, your decision to them. People who think outside their heads, the whole process of whose thought appears, like Homer's, in the act of secretion, who tell everything that led them towards this conclusion and away from that, ought never to be with the sick. *Conciseness necessary with sick.*

43 I have been told by women who had difficult confinements, that their strength depended upon the firmness of doctor and nurse. If either had betrayed that there was anything unusual or doubtful in the case, they felt it would have been "all over" with them. *And calmness.*

44 I have observed the same thing in acute cases, when the scale was trembling between life and death. If the doctor betrayed any want of decision, if the nurse lost any portion of her calmness or self-possession, it just turned the scale in favour of death.

45 Irresolution is what all patients most dread. Rather than meet this in others, they will collect all their data, and make up their *Irresolution most painful to them.*

52 Noise

minds for themselves. A change of mind in others, whether it is regarding an operation, or re-writing a letter, always injures the patient more than the being called upon to make up his mind to the most dreaded or difficult decision. Farther than this, in very many cases, the imagination in disease is far more active and vivid than it is in health. If you propose to the patient change of air to one place one hour, and to another the next, he has, in each case, immediately constituted himself in imagination the tenant of the place, gone over the whole premises in idea, and you have tired him as much by displacing his imagination, as if you had actually carried him over both places.

46 Above all leave the sick room quickly and come into it quickly, not suddenly, not with a rush. But don't let the patient be wearily waiting for when you will be out of the room or when you will be in it. Conciseness and decision in your movements, as well as your words, are necessary in the sick room, as necessary as absence of hurry and bustle. To possess yourself entirely will ensure you from either failing—either loitering or hurrying.

What a patient must not have to see to.

47 If a patient has to see, not only to his own but also to his nurse's punctuality, or perseverance, or readiness, or calmness, to any or all of these things, he is far better without that nurse than with her—however valuable and handy her services may otherwise be to him, and however incapable he may be of rendering them to himself.

Reading aloud.

48 With regard to reading aloud in the sick room, my experience is, that when the sick are too ill to read to themselves, they can seldom bear to be read to. Children, eye-patients, and uneducated persons are exceptions, or where there is any mechanical difficulty in reading. People who like to be read to, have generally not much the matter with them; while in fevers, or where there is much irritability of brain, the effort of listening to reading aloud has often brought on delirium. I speak with great diffidence; because there is an almost universal impression that it is *sparing* the sick to read aloud to them. But two things are certain:—

Read aloud slowly, distinctly, and steadily to the sick.

49 (1.) If there is some matter which *must* be read to a sick person, do it slowly. People often think that the way to get it over with least fatigue to him is to get it over in least time. They gabble; they plunge and gallop through the reading. There never was a greater mistake. Houdin, the conjuror, says that the way to make a story seem short

is to tell it slowly. So it is with reading to the sick. I have often heard a patient say to such a mistaken reader, "Don't read it to me; tell it me."* Unconsciously he is aware that this will regulate the plunging, the reading with unequal paces, slurring over one part, instead of leaving it out altogether, if it is unimportant, and mumbling another. If the reader lets his own attention wander, and then stops to read up to himself, or finds he has read the wrong bit, then it is all over with the poor patient's chance of not suffering. Very few people know how to read to the sick; very few read aloud as pleasantly even as they speak. In reading they sing, they hesitate, they stammer, they hurry, they mumble; when in speaking they do none of these things. Reading aloud to the sick ought always to be rather slow, and exceedingly distinct, but not mouthing—rather monotonous, but not sing song—rather loud, but not noisy—and above all, not too long. Be very sure of what your patient can bear.

50   (2.) The extraordinary habit of reading to one's-self in a sick room, and reading aloud to the patient any bits which will amuse him or more often the reader, is unaccountably thoughtless. What *do* you think the patient is thinking of during your gaps of non-reading? Do you think that he amuses himself upon what you have read for precisely the time it pleases you to go on reading to yourself, and that his attention is ready for something else at precisely the time it pleases you to begin reading again? Whether the person thus read to be sick or well, whether he be doing nothing or doing something else while being thus read to, the self-absorption and want of observation of the person who does it, is equally difficult to understand— although very often the read*ee* is too amiable to say how much it disturb him. Never read aloud by fits and starts to the sick.

51   One thing more:—From the flimsy manner in which most modern houses are built, where every step on the stairs, and along the floors, is felt all over the house; the higher the story, the greater the vibration. It is inconceivable how much the sick suffer by having anybody overhead. In the solidly built old houses, which, fortunately, most hospitals are, the noise and shaking is comparatively trifling. But it is a serious cause of suffering, in lightly built houses, and with the irritability peculiar to some diseases. Better far put such People overhead.

(49)   * Sick children, if not too shy to speak; will always express this wish. They invariably prefer a story to be told to them, rather than read to them. The sick would rather be told a thing than have it read to them.

patients at the top of the house, even with the additional fatigue of stairs, if you cannot secure the room above them being untenanted; you may otherwise bring on a state of restlessness which no opium will subdue. Do not neglect the warning, when a patient tells you that he "feels every step above him to cross his heart." Remember that every noise a patient cannot *see* partakes of the character of suddenness to him; and I am persuaded that patients with these peculiarly irritable nerves, are positively less injured by having persons in the same room with them than overhead, or separated by only a thin compartment. Any sacrifice to secure silence for these cases is worth while, because no air, however good, no attendance, however careful, will do anything for such cases without quiet.

<small>Music.</small>

52 The effect of music upon the sick has been scarcely at all noticed. In fact, its expensiveness, as it is now, makes any general application of it quite out of the question. I will only remark here, that wind instruments, including the human voice, and stringed instruments, capable of continuous sound, have generally a beneficent effect— while the piano-forte, with such instruments as have *no* continuity of sound, has just the reverse. The finest piano-forte playing will damage the sick, while an air, like "Home, sweet home," or "Assisa a piè d'un salice," on the most ordinary grinding organ will sensibly soothe them—and this quite independent of association.

53 Music, to the well, who *ought* to be active, gives the enjoyment of active life, without their having earned it. Music to the sick, who *cannot* be active, gives the enjoyment and takes away the nervous irritation of their incapacity.

V. VARIETY.

¹ To any but an old nurse, or an old patient, the degree would be quite inconceivable to which the nerves of the sick suffer from seeing the same walls, the same ceiling, the same surroundings during a long confinement to one or two rooms. Variety a means of recovery.

² **The superior cheerfulness of persons suffering severe paroxysms** of pain over that of persons suffering from nervous debility has often been remarked upon, and attributed to the enjoyment of the former of their intervals of respite. I incline to think that the majority of cheerful cases is to be found among those patients who are not confined to one room, whatever their suffering, and that the majority of depressed cases will be seen among those subjected to a long monotony of objects about them.

³ The nervous frame really suffers as much from this as the digestive organs from long monotony of diet, as *e.g.* the soldier from his twenty-one years' "boiled beef."

⁴ The effect in sickness of beautiful objects, of variety of objects, and especially of brilliancy of colour, is hardly at all appreciated. Colour and form means of recovery.

⁵ Such cravings are usually called the "fancies" of patients. And often doubtless patients have "fancies," as, *e.g.* when they desire two contradictions. But much more often, their (so-called) "fancies" are the most valuable indications of what is necessary for their recovery. And it would be well if nurses would watch these (so-called) "fancies" closely.

55

56 Variety

6   I have seen, in fevers (and felt, when I was a fever patient myself) the most acute suffering produced from the patient (in a hut) not being able to see out of window, and the knots in the wood being the only view. I shall never forget the rapture of fever patients over a bunch of bright-coloured flowers. I remember (in my own case) a nosegay of wild flowers being sent me, and from that moment recovery becoming more rapid.

<small>This is no fancy.</small>

7   People say the effect is only on the mind. It is no such thing. The effect is on the body, too. Little as we know about the way in which we are affected by form, by colour, and light, we do know this, that they have an actual physical effect.

8   Variety of form and brilliancy of colour in the objects presented to patients are actual means of recovery.

9   But it must be *slow* variety, *e.g.,* if you show a patient ten or twelve engravings successively, ten-to-one that he does not become cold and faint, or feverish, or even sick; but hang one up opposite him, one on each successive day, or week, or month, and he will revel in the variety.

<small>Flowers.</small>

10   The folly and ignorance which reign too often supreme over the sick room, cannot be better exemplified than by this. While the nurse will leave the patient stewing in a corrupting atmosphere, the best ingredient of which is carbonic acid; she will deny him, on the plea of unhealthiness, a glass of cut-flowers, or a growing plant. Now, no one ever saw "over-crowding" by plants in a room or ward. And the carbonic acid they give off at nights would not poison a fly. Nay, in overcrowded rooms, they actually absorb carbonic acid and give off oxygen. Cut-flowers also decompose water and produce oxygen gas. It is true there are certain flowers, *e.g.,* lilies, the smell of which is said to depress the nervous system. These are easily known by the smell, and can be avoided.

<small>Effect of body on mind.</small>

11   Volumes are now written and spoken upon the effect of the mind upon the body. Much of it is true. But I wish a little more was thought of the effect of the body on the mind. You who believe yourselves overwhelmed with anxieties, but are able every day to walk up Regent-street, or out in the country, to take your meals with others in other room, &c., &c., you little know how much **your** anxieties are thereby lightened; you little know how intensified they become to those who can have no change; how the very walls of their sick rooms seem

hung with their cares; how the ghosts of their troubles haunt their beds; how impossible it is for them to escape from a pursuing thought without some help from variety.

12   It is a matter of painful wonder to the sick themselves how much painful ideas predominate over pleasurable ones in their impressions; they reason with themselves; they think themselves ungrateful; it is all of no use. The fact is, that these painful impressions are far better dismissed by a real laugh, if you can excite one by books or conversation, than by any direct reasoning; or if the patient is too weak to laugh, some impression from nature is what he wants. I have mentioned the cruelty of letting him stare at a dead wall. In many diseases, especially in convalescence from fever, that wall will appear to make all sorts of faces at him; now flowers never do this. Form, colour, will free your patient from his painful ideas better than any argument. *(Sick suffer to excess from mental as well as bodily pain.)*

13   A patient can just as much move his leg when it is fractured as change his thoughts when no external help from variety is given him. This is, indeed, one of the main sufferings of sickness; just as the fixed posture is one of the main sufferings of the broken limb.

14   It is an ever recurring wonder to see educated people, who call themselves nurses, acting thus. They vary their own objects, their own employments, many times a day; and while nursing (!) some bed-ridden sufferer, they let him lie there staring at a dead wall, without any change of object to enable him to vary his thoughts; and it never even occurs to them, at least to move his bed so that he can look out of window. No, the bed is to be always left in the darkest, dullest, remotest, part of the room. *(Help the sick to vary their thoughts.)*

15   I remember a case in point. A man received an injury to the spine, from an accident, which after a long confinement ended in death. He was a workman—had not in his composition a single grain of what is called "enthusiasm for nature"—but he was desperate to "see once more out of window." His nurse actually got him on her back, and managed to perch him up at the window for an instant, "to see out." The consequence to the poor nurse was a serious illness, which nearly proved fatal. The man never knew it; but a great many other people did. Yet the consequence in none of their minds, so far as I know, was the conviction that the craving for variety in the starving eye is just as desperate as that for food in the starving *(Desperate desire in the sick to "see out of window.")*

58 Variety

stomach, and tempts the famishing creature in either case to steal for its satisfaction. No other word will express it but "desperation." And it sets the seal of ignorance and stupidity just as much on the governors and attendants of the sick if they do not provide the sick-bed with a "view," or with variety of some kind, as if they did not provide the hospital with a kitchen.

16 And in no case does consideration of these matters meet with the same success as it does for the sick. Poets rave about the "charms of nature." I question whether the intensest pleasure ever felt in nature is not that of the sick man raising a forest tree, six inches high, from an acorn or a horse-chestnut, in a London back-court. Europe perhaps never gives such during a life-long travel.

17 It is a very common error among the well to think that "with a little more self-control" the sick might, if they choose, "dismiss painful thoughts" which "aggravate their disease," &c. Believe me, almost *any* sick person, who behaves decently well, exercises more self-control every moment of his day than you will ever know till you are sick yourself. Almost every step that crosses his room is painful to him; almost every thought that crosses his brain is painful to him; and if he can speak without being savage, and look without being unpleasant, he is exercising self-control.

18 Suppose you have been up all night, and instead of being allowed to have your cup of tea, you were to be told that you ought to "exercise self-control," what should you say? Now, the nerves of the sick are always in the state that yours are in after you have been up all night.

Supply to the sick the defect of manual labour.

19 We will suppose the diet of the sick to be cared for. Then, this state of nerves is most frequently to be relieved by care in affording them a pleasant view, a judicious variety as to flowers,* and pretty things. Light by itself will often relieve it. The craving for "the return of day," which the sick so constantly evince, is generally nothing but the desire for light, the remembrance of the relief which a variety of objects before the eye affords to the harassed sick mind.

20 Again, every man and every woman has some amount of manual employment, excepting a few fine ladies, who do not even dress themselves, and who are virtually in the same category, as to nerves, as

Physical effect of colour.

(19) * No one who has watched the sick can doubt the fact, that some feel stimulus from looking at scarlet flowers, exhaustion from looking at deep blue, &c.

the sick. Now, you can have no idea of the relief which manual labour is to you—of the degree to which the deprivation of manual employment increases the peculiar irritability from which many sick suffer.

21   A little needle-work, a little writing, a little cleaning, would be the greatest relief the sick could have, if they could do it; these *are* the greatest relief to you, though you do not know it. Reading, though it is often the only thing the sick can do, is not this relief. Bearing this in mind, bearing in mind that you have all these varieties of employment which the sick cannot have, bear also in mind to obtain for them all the varieties which they can enjoy.

22   I need hardly say that excess in needle-work, in writing, in any other continuous employment, will produce the same irritability that defect in manual employment (as one cause) produces in the sick.

VI. TAKING FOOD.

¹ Every careful observer of the sick will agree in this that thousands of patients are annually starved in the midst of plenty, from want of attention to the ways which alone make it possible for them to take food. This want of attention is as remarkable in those who urge upon the sick to do what is quite impossible to them, as in the sick themselves who will not make the effort to do what is perfectly possible to them.

<small>Want of attention to hours of taking food.</small>

² For instance, to the large majority of very weak patients it is quite impossible to take any solid food before 11 a.m., nor then, if their strength is still further exhausted by fasting till that hour. For weak patients have generally feverish nights and, in the morning, dry mouths; and, if they could eat with those dry mouths, it would be the worse for them. A spoonful of beef-tea, of arrowroot and wine, of egg flip, every hour, will give them the requisite nourishment, and prevent them from being too much exhausted to take at a later hour the solid food, which is necessary for their recovery. And every patient who can swallow at all can swallow these liquid things, if he chooses. But how often do we hear a mutton-chop, an egg, a bit of bacon, ordered to a patient for breakfast, to whom (as a moment's consideration would show us) it must be quite impossible to masticate such things at that hour.

³ Again, a nurse is ordered to give a patient a tea-cup full of some article of food every three hours. The patient's stomach rejects it.

If so, try a table-spoon full every hour; if this will not do, a tea-spoon full every quarter of an hour.

4   I am bound to say, that I think more patients are lost by want of care and ingenuity in these momentous minutiæ in private nursing than in public hospitals. And I think there is more of the *entente cordiale* to assist one another's hands between the doctor and his head nurse in the latter institutions, than between the doctor and the patient's friends in the private house.

<small>Life often hangs upon minutes in taking food.</small>

5   If we did but know the consequences which may ensue, in very weak patients, from ten minutes' fasting or repletion (I call it repletion when they are obliged to let too small an interval elapse between taking food and some other exertion, owing to the nurse's unpunctuality), we should be more careful never to let this occur. In very weak patients there is often a nervous difficulty of swallowing, which is so much increased by any other call upon their strength that, unless they have their food punctually at the minute, which minute again must be arranged so as to fall in with no other minute's occupation, they can take nothing till the next respite occurs—so that an unpunctuality or delay of ten minutes may very well turn out to be one of two or three hours. And why is it not as easy to be punctual to a minute? Life often literally hangs upon these minutes.

6   In acute cases, where life or death is to be determined in a few hours, these matters are very generally attended to, especially in Hospitals; and the number of cases is large where the patient is, as it were, brought back to life by exceeding care on the part of the Doctor or Nurse, or both, in ordering and giving nourishment with minute selection and punctuality.

<small>Patients often starved in chronic cases.</small>

7   But, in chronic cases, lasting over months and years, where the fatal issue is often determined at last by mere protracted starvation, I had rather not enumerate the instances which I have known where a little ingenuity, and a great deal of perseverance, might, in all probability, have averted the result. The consulting the hours when the patient can take food, the observation of the times, often varying, when he is most faint, the altering seasons of taking food, in order to anticipate and prevent such times—all this, which requires observation, ingenuity, and perseverance (and these really constitute the good Nurse), might save more lives than we wot of.

<small>Food never to be left by the patient's side.</small>

8   To leave the patient's untasted food by his side, from meal to

meal, in hopes that he will eat it in the interval, is simply to prevent him from taking any food at all. Patients have been literally incapacitated from taking one article of food after another, by this piece of ignorance. Let the food come at the right time, and be taken away, eaten or uneaten, at the right time; but never let a patient have "something always standing" by him, if you don't wish to disgust him of everything.

9. On the other hand, a patient's life has been saved (he was sinking for want of food), by the simple question, put to him by the doctor, "But is there no hour when you feel you could eat?" "Oh, yes," he said, "I could always take something at — o'clock and — o'clock." The thing was tried and succeeded. Patients very seldom, however, can tell this; it is for you to watch and find it out.

10. A patient should, if possible, not see or smell either the food of others, or a greater amount of food than he himself can consume at one time, or even hear food talked about or see it in the raw state. I know of no exception to the above rule. The breaking of it always induces a greater or less incapacity of taking food.

Patient had better not see more food than his own.

11. In hospital wards it is of course impossible to observe all this; and in single wards, where a patient must be continuously and closely watched, it is frequently impossible to relieve the attendant, so that his or her own meals can be taken out of the ward. But it is not the less true that, in such cases, even where the patient is not himself aware of it, his possibility of taking food is limited by seeing the attendant eating meals under his observation. In some cases the sick are aware of it, and complain. A case where the patient was supposed to be insensible, but complained as soon as able to speak, is now present to my recollection.

12. Remember, however, that the extreme punctuality in well-ordered hospitals, the rule that nothing shall be done in the ward while the patients are having their meals, go far to counterbalance what unavoidable evil there is in having patients together. The private nurse may be often seen dusting or fidgeting about in a sick room all the while the patient is eating, or trying to eat.

13. That the more alone an invalid can be when taking food, the better, is unquestionable; and, even if he must be fed, the nurse should not allow him to talk, or talk to him, especially about food, while eating.

14. When a person is compelled, by the pressure of occupation, to

continue his business while sick, it ought to be a rule without any exception whatever, that no one shall bring business to him or talk to him while he is taking food, nor go on talking to him on interesting subjects up to the last moment before his meals, nor make an engagement with him immediately after, so that there be any hurry of mind while taking them.

15   Upon the observance of these rules, especially the first, often depends the patient's capability of taking food at all, or, if he is amiable and forces himself to take food, of deriving any nourishment from it.

<small>You cannot be too careful as to quality in sick diet.</small>

16   A nurse should never put before a patient milk that is sour, meat or soup that is turned, an egg that is bad, or vegetables underdone. Yet often these things are brought in to the sick in a state perfectly perceptible to every nose or eye except the nurse's. It is here that the clever nurse appears; she will not bring in the peccant article, but, not to disappoint the patient, she will whip up something else in a few minutes. Remember that sick cookery should half do the work of your poor patient's weak digestion. But if you further impair it with your bad articles, I know not what is to become of him or of it.

17   If the nurse is an intelligent being, and not a mere carrier of diets to and from the patient, let her exercise her intelligence in these things. How often have we known a patient eat nothing at all in the day, because one meal was left untasted (at that time he was incapable of eating), at another the milk was sour, the third was spoiled by some other accident. And it never occurred to the nurse to extemporize some expedient,—it never occurred to her that as he had had no solid food that day, he might eat a bit of toast (say) with his tea in the evening, or he might have some meal an hour earlier. A patient who cannot touch his dinner at two, will often accept it gladly, if brought to him at seven. But somehow nurses never "think of these things." One would imagine they did not consider themselves bound to exercise their judgment; they leave it to the patient. Now I am quite sure that it is better for a patient rather to suffer these neglects than to try to teach his nurse to nurse him, if she does not know how. It ruffles him, and if he is ill he is in no condition to teach, especially upon himself. The above remarks apply much more to private nursing than to hospitals.

<small>Nurse must have some rule of thought about her patient's diet.</small>

18   I would say to the nurse, have a rule of thought about your patient's

diet; consider, remember how much he has had, and how much he ought to have to-day. Generally, the only rule of the private patient's diet is what the nurse has to give. It is true she cannot give him what she has not got; but his stomach does not wait for her convenience, or even her necessity. If it is used to having its stimulus at one hour to-day, and to-morrow it does not have it, because she has failed in getting it, he will suffer. She must be always exercising her ingenuity to supply defects, and to remedy accidents which will happen among the best contrivers, but from which the patient does not suffer the less, because "they cannot be helped."

19 Why, because the nurse has not got some food to-day which the patient takes, can the patient wait four hours for it to-day, who could not wait two hours yesterday? Yet this is the only logic one generally hears. On the other hand, the opposite course, viz., of the nurse giving the patient a thing because she *has* got it, is equally fatal. If she happens to have fresh jelly, or fresh fruit, she will frequently give it to the patient half-an-hour after his dinner, or at his dinner, when he cannot possibly eat that and the broth too—or, worse still, leave it by his bed-side till he is so sickened with the sight of it, that he cannot eat it at all. *Nurse must have some rule of time about the patient's diet.*

20 One very minute caution,—take care not to spill into your patient's saucer, in other words, take care that the outside bottom rim of his cup is quite dry and clean; if, every time he lifts his cup to his lips, he has to carry the saucer with it, or else to drop the liquid upon and to soil his sheet, or his bed-gown, or pillow, or, if he is sitting up, his dress, you have no idea what a difference this minute want of care on your part makes to his comfort and even to his willingness for food. *Keep your patient's cup dry underneath.*

VII. WHAT FOOD?

1   I will mention one or two of the most common errors among women in charge of sick respecting sick diet. One is the belief that beef tea is the most nutritive of all articles. Now, just try and boil down a lb. of beef into beef tea, evaporate your beef tea, and see what is left of your beef. You will find that there is barely a teaspoonful of solid nourishment to half-a-pint of water in beef tea;—nevertheless there is a certain reparative quality in it, we do not know what, as there is in tea;—but it may safely be given in almost any inflammatory disease, and is as little to be depended upon with the healthy or convalescent as where much nourishment is required. Again, it is an ever ready saw that an egg is equivalent to a lb. of meat,—whereas it is not at all so. Also, it is seldom noticed with how many patients, particularly of nervous or bilious temperament, eggs disagree. All puddings made with eggs, are distasteful to them in consequence. An egg, whipped up with wine, is often the only form in which they can take this kind of nourishment. Again, if the patient has attained to eating meat, it is supposed that to give him meat is the only thing needful for his recovery; whereas scorbutic sores have been actually known to appear among sick persons living in the midst of plenty in England, which could be traced to no other source than this, viz.: that the nurse, depending on meat alone, had allowed the patient to be without vegetables for a considerable time, these latter being so badly cooked that he always left them untouched. Arrowroot

Common errors in diet.

Beef tea.

Eggs.

Meat without vegetables.

Arrowroot.

68 What Food?

is another grand dependence of the nurse. As a vehicle for wine, and as a restorative quickly prepared, it is all very well. But it is nothing but starch and water. Flour is both more nutritive, and less liable to ferment, and is preferable wherever it can be used.

<small>Milk, butter, cream, &c.</small>

2   Again, milk and the preparations from milk, are a most important article of food for the sick. Butter is the lightest kind of animal fat, and though it wants the sugar and some of the other elements which there are in milk, yet it is most valuable both in itself and in enabling the patient to eat more bread. Flour, oats, groats, barley, and their kind, are as we have already said, preferable in all their preparations to all the preparations of arrowroot, sago, tapioca, and their kind. Cream, in many long chronic diseases, is quite irreplaceable by any other article whatever. It seems to act in the same manner as beef tea, and to most it is much easier of digestion than milk. In fact, it seldom disagrees. Cheese is not usually digestible by the sick, but it is pure nourishment for repairing waste; and I have seen sick, and not a few either, whose craving for cheese showed how much it was needed by them.*

3   But, if fresh milk is so valuable a food for the sick, the least change or sourness in it, makes it of all articles, perhaps, the most injurious; diarrhoea is a common result of fresh milk allowed to become at all sour. The nurse therefore ought to exercise her utmost care in this. In large institutions for the sick, even the poorest, the utmost care is exercised. Wenham Lake ice is used for this express purpose every summer, while the private patient, perhaps, never tastes a drop of milk that is not sour, all through the hot weather, so little does the private nurse understand the necessity of such care. Yet, if you consider that the only drop of real nourishment in your patient's tea is the drop of milk, and how much almost all English patients depend upon their tea, you will see the great importance of not depriving your patient of this drop of milk. Buttermilk, a totally

<small>(2) Intelligent cravings of particular sick for particular articles of diet.</small>

* In the diseases produced by bad food, such as scorbutic dysentery and diarrhœa, the patient's stomach often craves for and digests things, some of which certainly would be laid down in no dietary that ever was invented for sick, and especially not for such sick. These are fruit, pickles, jams, gingerbread, fat of ham or of bacon, suet, cheese, butter, milk. These cases I have seen not by ones, nor by tens, but by hundreds. And the patient's stomach was right and the book was wrong. The articles craved for, in these cases, might have been principally arranged under the two heads of fat and vegetable acids.

There is often a marked difference between men and women in this matter of sick feeding. Women's digestion is generally slower.

different thing, is often very useful, especially in fevers.

4   In laying down rules of diet, by the amounts of "solid nutriment" in different kinds of food, it is constantly lost sight of what the patient requires to repair his waste, what he can take and what he can't. You cannot diet a patient from a book, you cannot make up the human body as you would make up a prescription,—so many parts "carboniferous," so many parts "nitrogenous" will constitute a perfect diet for the patient. The nurse's observation here will materially assist the doctor—the patient's "fancies" will materially assist the nurse. For instance, sugar is one of the most nutritive of all articles, being pure carbon, and is particularly recommended in some books. But the vast majority of all patients in England, young and old, male and female, rich and poor, hospital and private, dislike sweet things,— and while I have never known a person take to sweets when he was ill who disliked them when he was well, I have known many fond of them when in health, who in sickness would leave off anything sweet, even to sugar in tea,—sweet puddings, sweet drinks, are their aversion; the furred tongue almost always likes what is sharp or pungent. Scorbutic patients are an exception, they often crave for sweetmeats and jams. *Sweet things.*

5   Jelly is another article of diet in great favour with nurses and friends of the sick; even if it could be eaten solid, it would not nourish, but it is simply the height of folly to take $\frac{1}{8}$ oz. of gelatine and make it into a certain bulk by dissolving it in water and then to give it to the sick, as if the mere bulk represented nourishment. It is now known that jelly does not nourish, that it has a tendency to produce diarrhœa,—and to trust to it to repair the waste of a diseased constitution is simply to starve the sick under the guise of feeding them. If one hundred spoonfuls of jelly were given in the course of the day, you would have given one spoonful of gelatine, which spoonful has no nutritive power whatever. *Jelly.*

6   And, nevertheless, gelatine contains a large quantity of nitrogen, which is one of the most powerful elements in nutrition; on the other hand, beef tea may be chosen as an illustration of great nutrient power in sickness, co-existing with a very small amount of solid nitrogenous matter.

7   Dr. Christison says that "every one will be struck with the readiness with which" certain classes of "patients will often take diluted *Beef tea.*

meat juice or beef tea repeatedly, when they refuse all other kinds of food." This is particularly remarkable in "cases of gastric fever, in which," he says, "little or nothing else besides beef tea or diluted meat juice" has been taken for weeks or even months; 'and yet a pint of beef tea contains scarcely $\frac{1}{4}$ oz. of anything but water.'"—The result is so striking that he asks what is its mode of action? "Not simply nutrient— $\frac{1}{4}$ oz. of the most nutritive material cannot nearly replace the daily wear and tear of the tissues in any circumstances. Possibly," he says, "it belongs to a new denomination of remedies."

8   It has been observed that a small quantity of beef tea added to other articles of nutrition augments their power out of all proportion to the additional amount of solid matter.

9   The reason why jelly should be innutritious and beef tea nutritious to the sick, is a secret yet undiscovered, but it clearly shows that careful observation of the sick is the only clue to the best dietary.

<small>Observation, not chemistry, must decide sick diet.</small>

10   Chemistry has as yet afforded little insight into the dieting of the sick. All that chemistry can tell us is the amount of "carboniferous" or "nitrogenous" elements discoverable in different dietetic articles. It has given us lists of dietetic substances, arranged in the order of their richness in one or other of these principles; but that is all. In the great majority of cases, the stomach of the patient is guided by other principles of selection than merely the amount of carbon or nitrogen in the diet. No doubt, in this as in other things, nature has very definite rules for her guidance, but these rules can only be ascertained by the most careful observation at the bed-side. She there teaches us that living chemistry, the chemistry of reparation, is something different from the chemistry of the laboratory. Organic chemistry is useful, as all knowledge is, when we come face to face with nature; but it by no means follows that we should learn in the laboratory any one of the reparative processes going on in disease.

11   Again, the nutritive power of milk and of the preparations from milk, is very much undervalued; there is nearly as much nourishment in half a pint of milk as there is in a quarter of a lb. of meat. But this is not the whole question or nearly the whole. The main question is, what the patient's stomach can assimilate or derive nourishment from, and of this the patient's stomach is the sole judge. Chemistry cannot tell this. The patient's stomach must be its own

chemist. The diet which will keep the healthy man healthy, will kill the sick one. The same beef which is the most nutritive of all meat, and which nourishes the healthy man, is the least nourishing of all food to the sick man, whose half-dead stomach can *assimilate* no part of it, that is, make no food out of it. On a diet of beef tea healthy men on the other hand speedily lose their strength.

12   I have known patients live for many months without touching bread, because they could not eat baker's bread. These were mostly country patients, but not all. Home-made bread or brown bread is a most important article of diet for many patients. The use of aperients may be entirely superseded by it. Oat cake is another. *(Home-made bread.)*

13   To watch for the opinions, then, which the patient's stomach gives, rather than to read "analyses of foods," is the business of all those who have to settle what the patient is to eat—perhaps the most important thing to be provided for him after the air he is to breathe. *(Sound observation has scarcely yet been brought to bear on sick diet.)*

14   Now the medical man who sees the patient only once a day, or even only once or twice a week, cannot possibly tell this without the assistance of the patient himself, or of those who are in constant observation of the patient. The utmost the medical man can tell is whether the patient is weaker or stronger at this visit than he was at the last visit. I should therefore say that incomparably the most important office of the nurse, after she has taken care of the patient's air, is to take care to observe the effect of his food, and report it to the medical attendant.

15   It is quite incalculable the good that would certainly come from such *sound* and close observation in this almost neglected branch of nursing, or the help it would give to the medical man.

16   A great deal too much against tea is said by wise people, and a great deal too much of tea is given to the sick by foolish people. When you see the natural and almost universal craving in English sick for their "tea," you cannot but feel that nature knows what she is about. But a little tea or coffee restores them quite as much as a great deal, and a great deal of tea and especially of coffee impairs the little power of digestion they have. Yet a nurse because she sees how one or two cups of tea or coffee restores her patient, thinks that three or four cups will do twice as much. This is not the case at all; it is however certain that there is nothing yet discovered which is a substitute to the English patient for his cup of tea; he can take it when *(Tea and coffee.)*

he can take nothing else, and he often can't take anything else if he has it not. I should be very glad if any of the abusers of tea would point out what to give to an English patient after a sleepless night, instead of tea. If you give it at five or six o'clock in the morning, he may even sometimes fall asleep after it, and get perhaps his only two or three hours' sleep during the twenty-four. At the same time you never should give tea or coffee to the sick, as a rule, after five o'clock in the afternoon. Sleeplessness in the early night is from excitement generally and is increased by tea or coffee; sleeplessness which continues to the early morning is from exhaustion often, and is relieved by tea. The only English patients I have ever known refuse tea, have been typhus cases, and the first sign of their getting better was their craving again for tea. In general, the dry and dirty tongue always prefers tea to coffee, and will quite decline milk, unless with tea. Coffee is a better restorative than tea, but a greater impairer of the digestion. Let the patient's taste decide. You will say that, in cases of great thirst, the patient's craving decides that it will drink *a great deal* of tea, and that you cannot help it. But in these cases be sure that the patient requires diluents for quite other purposes than quenching the thirst; he wants a great deal of some drink, not only of tea, and the doctor will order what he is to have, barley water or lemonade, or soda water and milk, as the case may be.

17   It is made a frequent recommendation to persons about to incur great exhaustion, either from the nature of the service or from their being not in a state fit for it, to eat a piece of bread before they go. I wish the recommenders would themselves try the experiment of substituting a piece of bread for a cup of tea or coffee or beef tea as a refresher. They would find it a very poor comfort. When soldiers have to set out fasting on fatiguing duty, when nurses have to go fasting in to their patients, it is a hot restorative they want, and ought to have, before they go, not a cold bit of bread. And dreadful have been the consequences of neglecting this. If they can take a bit of bread *with* the hot cup of tea, so much the better, but not *instead* of it. The fact that there is more nourishment in bread than in almost anything else has probably induced the mistake. That it is a fatal mistake there is no doubt. It seems, though very little is known on the subject, that what "assimilates" itself directly and with the least trouble of

digestion with the human body is the best for the above circumstances. Bread requires two or three processes of assimilation, before it becomes like the human body.

18 The almost universal testimony of English men and women who have undergone great fatigue, such as riding long journeys without stopping, or sitting up for several nights in succession, is that they could do it best upon an occasional cup of tea—and nothing else.

19 Let experience, not theory, decide upon this as upon all other things.

20 Lehmann, quoted by Dr. Christison, says that, among the well and active "the infusion of 1 oz. of roasted coffee daily will diminish the waste" going on in the body "by one-fourth," and Dr. Christison adds that tea has the same property. Now this is actual experiment. Lehmann weighs the man and finds the fact from his weight. It is not deduced from any "analysis" of food. All experience among the sick shows the same thing.

21 In making coffee for the sick, it is absolutely necessary to buy it in the berry and grind it at home. Otherwise you may reckon upon its containing a certain amount of chicory, *at least*. This is not a question of the taste or of the wholesomeness of chicory. It is that chicory has nothing at all of the properties for which you give coffee. And therefore you may as well not give it.

22 Again, all laundresses, mistresses of dairy-farms, head nurses (I speak of the good old sort only—women who unite a good deal of hard manual labour with the head-work necessary for arranging the day's business, so that none of it shall tread upon the heels of something else) set great value, I have observed, upon having a high-priced tea. This is called extravagant. But these women are "extravagant" in nothing else. And they are right in this. Real tea-leaf tea alone contains the restorative they want; which is not to be found in sloe-leaf tea.

23 The mistresses of houses, who cannot even go over their own house once a-day, are incapable of judging for these women. For they are incapable themselves, to all appearance, of the spirit of arrangement (no small task) necessary for managing a large ward or dairy.

24 Cocoa is often recommended to the sick in lieu of tea or coffee. But independently of the fact that English sick very generally dislike cocoa, it has quite a different effect from tea or coffee. It is an oily

Cocoa.

74 What Food?

starchy nut, having no restorative power at all, but simply increasing fat. It is pure mockery of the sick, therefore, to call it a substitute for tea. For any renovating stimulus it has, you might just as well offer them chestnuts instead of tea.

Bulk.   25   An almost universal error among nurses is in the bulk of the food and especially the drinks they offer to their patients. Suppose a patient ordered four oz. brandy during the day, how is he to take this if you make it into four pints with diluting it? The same with tea and beef tea, with arrowroot, milk, &c. You have not increased the nourishment, you have not increased the renovating power of these articles, by increasing their bulk,—you have very likely diminished both by giving the patient's digestion more to do, and, most likely of all, the patient will leave half of what he has been ordered to take, because he cannot swallow the bulk with which you have been pleased to invest it. It requires very nice observation and care (and meets with hardly any) to determine what will not be too thick or strong for the patient to take, while giving him no more than the bulk which he is able to swallow.

VIII. BED AND BEDDING.

¹ A few words upon bedsteads and bedding; and principally as regards patients who are entirely, or almost entirely, confined to bed.

² Feverishness is generally supposed to be a symptom of fever— in nine cases out of ten it is a symptom of bedding.

³ The patient has had re-introduced into the body the emanations from himself which day after day and week after week saturate his unaired bedding. How can it be otherwise? Look at the ordinary bed in which a patient lies.

⁴ If I were looking out for an example in order to show what *not* to do, I should take the specimen of an ordinary bed in a private house: a wooden bedstead, two or even three mattresses piled up to above the height of a table; a vallance attached to the frame—nothing but a miracle could ever thoroughly dry or air such a bed and bedding. The patient must inevitably alternate between cold damp after his bed is made, and warm damp before, both saturated with organic matter, and this from the time the mattresses are put under him till the time they are picked to pieces, if this is ever done.

⁵ For the same reason, if, after washing a patient, you must put the same night-dress on him again, always give it a preliminary warm at the fire. The night-gown he has worn must be, to a certain extent, damp. It has now got cold from having been off him for a few minutes. The fire will dry and at the same time air it. This is much

Marginalia:
- (¶1) Feverishness a symptom of bedding.
- (¶4) Uncleanliness of ordinary bedding.

76 Bed & Bedding

6   If you consider that an adult in health exhales by the lungs and skin in the twenty-four hours three pints at least of moisture, loaded with organic matter ready to enter into putrefaction; that in sickness the quantity is often greatly increased, the quality is always more noxious—just ask yourself next where does all this moisture go to? Chiefly into the bedding, because it cannot go anywhere else. And it stays there; because, except perhaps a weekly change of sheets, scarcely any other airing is attempted. A nurse will be careful to fidgetiness about airing the clean sheets from clean damp, but airing the dirty sheets from noxious damp will never even occur to her. Besides this, the most dangerous effluvia we know of are from the excreta of the sick—these are placed, at least temporarily, where they must throw their effluvia into the under side of the bed, and the space under the bed is never aired; it cannot be, with our arrangements. Must not such a bed be always saturated, and be always the means of re-introducing into the system of the unfortunate patient who lies in it, that excrementitious matter to eliminate which from the body nature had expressly appointed the disease?

Air your dirty sheets, not only your clean ones.

7   My heart always sinks within me when I hear the good housewife, of every class, say, "I assure you the bed has been well slept in," and one can only hope it is not true. What? is the bed already saturated with somebody else's damp before my patient comes to exhale into it his own damp? Has it not had a single chance to be aired? No, not one. "It has been slept in every night."

8   The only way of really nursing a real patient is to have an *iron* bedstead, with rheocline springs, which are permeable by the air up to the very mattress (no vallance, of course), the mattress to be a thin hair one; the bed to be not above $3\frac{1}{2}$ feet wide. If the patient be entirely confined to his bed, there should be *two* such bedsteads; each bed to be "made" with mattress, sheets, blankets, &c., complete—the patient to pass twelve hours in each bed; on no account to carry his sheets with him. The whole of the bedding to be hung up to air for each intermediate twelve hours. Of course there are many cases where this cannot be done at all—many more where only an approach to it can be made. I am indicating the ideal of nursing, and what has actually been done. But about the kind of bedstead there can be no doubt, whether there be one or two provided.

Iron spring bedstead the best.

Comfort and cleanliness of two beds.

9   There is a prejudice in favour of a wide bed—I believe it to be a prejudice. All the refreshment of moving a patient from one side to the other of his bed is far more effectually secured by putting him into a fresh bed; and a patient who is really very ill does not stray far in bed. But it is said there is no room to put a tray down on a narrow bed. No good nurse will ever put a tray on a bed at all. If the patient can turn on his side, he will eat more comfortably from a bed-side table; and on no account whatever should a bed ever be higher than a sofa. Otherwise the patient feels himself "out of humanity's reach"; he can get at nothing for himself: he can move nothing for himself. If the patient cannot turn, a table over the bed is a better thing. I need hardly say that a patient's bed should never have its side against the wall. The nurse must be able to get easily to both sides of the bed, and to reach easily every part of the patient without stretching—a thing impossible if the bed be either too wide or too high. *(Bed not to be too wide.)*

10   When I see a patient in a room nine or ten feet high upon a bed between four and five feet high, with his head, when he is sitting up in bed, actually within two or three feet of the ceiling, I ask myself, is this expressly planned to produce that peculiarly distressing feeling common to the sick, viz., as if the walls and ceiling were closing in upon them, and they becoming sandwiches between floor and ceiling, which imagination is not, indeed, here so far from the truth? If, over and above this, the window stops short of the ceiling, then the patient's head may literally be raised above the stratum of fresh air, even when the window is open. Can human perversity any farther go, in unmaking the process of restoration which God has made? The fact is, that the heads of sleepers or of sick should never be higher than the throat of the chimney, which ensures their being in the current of best air. And we will not suppose it possible that you have closed your chimney with a chimney-board. *(Bed not to be too high.)*

11   If a bed is higher than a sofa, the difference of the fatigue of getting in and out of bed will just make the difference, very often, to the patient (who can get in and out of bed at all) of being able to take a few minutes exercise, either in the open air or in another room. It is so very odd that people never think of this, or of how many more times a patient who is in bed for the twenty-four hours is obliged to get in and out of bed than they are, who only, it is to be hoped, get

78 Bed & Bedding

into bed once and out of bed once during the twenty-four hours.

Nor in a dark place.

12   A patient's bed should always be in the lightest spot in the room; and he should be able to see out of window.

Nor a four poster with curtains.

13   I need scarcely say that the old four-post bed with curtains is utterly inadmissible, whether for sick or well. Hospital bedsteads are in many respects very much less objectionable than private ones.

Scrofula often a result of disposition of bedclothes.

14   There is reason to believe that not a few of the apparently unaccountable cases of scrofula among children proceed from the habit of sleeping with the head under the bed clothes, and so inhaling air already breathed, which is farther contaminated by exhalations from the skin. Patients are sometimes given to a similar habit, and it often happens that the bed clothes are so disposed that the patient must necessarily breathe air more or less contaminated by exhalations from his skin. A good nurse will be careful to attend to this. It is an important part, so to speak, of ventilation.

15   Consumptive patients often put their heads under the bed clothes, because it relieves a paroxysm of coughing, brought on by a change of temperature or of moisture in our changeable atmosphere. Of all places to take warm air from, one's own body is certainly the worst. And perhaps, if nurses do encourage this practice, we need no longer wonder at the "rapid decline" of some consumptive patients. A folded silk handkerchief, lightly laid over the mouth, a respirator, medicated inhalations, or merely inhaling the steam from a basin of boiling water, will relieve the paroxysm of coughing without such danger. But inhalations must be carefully managed, so as not to make the patient damp.

Bed sores.

16   It may be worth while to remark, that where there is any danger of bed-sores a blanket should never be placed *under* the patient. It retains damp and acts like a poultice.

Heavy and impervious bedclothes.

17   Never use anything but light Witney blankets as bed covering for the sick. The heavy cotton impervious counterpane is bad, for the very reason that it keeps in the emanations from the sick person, while the blanket allows them to pass through. Weak patients are invariably distressed by a great weight of bed-clothes, which often prevents their getting any sound sleep whatever.

Nurses often do not think the sick-room any business of theirs, but only the sick.

18   I once told a "very good nurse" that the way in which her patient's room was kept was quite enough to account for his sleeplessness; and she answered with perfect good-humour that she was not at all

surprised at it—as if the state of the room were, like the state of the weather, entirely out of her power. Now in what sense was this woman to be called a "nurse?"

19   A true nurse will always make her patient's bed herself, not leave it to the housemaid. In well-managed hospital wards, the head nurse (or "sister") makes the beds of the worst cases herself, and is always the best bed-maker in the ward. If you consider the importance of sleep to the sick, the necessity of a well-made bed to procure them sleep, you will not leave this essential part of your functions to *any* one. But a careless nurse doubles the blankets over the patient's chest, instead of leaving the lightest weight there—she puts a thick warm blanket under him—she does not turn his mattress everyway *every* day; and the patient would rather than not that his bed were made by anybody else.

20   One word about pillows. Every weak patient, be his illness what it may, suffers more or less, from difficulty in breathing. (1.) To take the weight of the body off the poor chest, which is hardly up to its work as it is, ought therefore to be the object of the nurse in arranging his pillows. Now what does she do and what are the consequences? She piles the pillows one a-top of the other like a wall of bricks. The head is thrown upon the chest. And the shoulders are pushed forward, so as not to allow the lungs room to expand. The pillows, in fact, lean upon the patient, not the patient upon the pillows. It is impossible to give a rule for this, because it must vary with the figure of the patient. But the object is to support, with the pillows, the back *below* the breathing apparatus, to allow the shoulders room to fall back, and to support the head, without throwing it forward. The suffering of dying patients is immensely increased by neglect of these points. And many an invalid, too weak to drag about his pillows himself, slips his book or anything at hand behind the lower part of his back to support it. (2.) Tall patients suffer much more than short ones, because of the *drag* of the long limbs upon the waist. Something to press the feet against is a relief to all.

Pillows.

21   Having said this about the two principles to be observed for giving ease to patients in bed, I must add that they apply equally to them when up. I scarcely ever saw an invalid chair which was not constructed in express violation of both—which did not, that is, *increase* the drag of the limbs upon the waist, and throw too much of the weight

Invalid chairs.

upon the axis of the spine, thereby preventing any relief to the chest. An ordinary *low* well-stuffed arm-chair with pillows and a footstool is generally far better than any of the elaborate invalid chairs. The very idea of mounting into one of them terrifies a patient. They are all too high, too deep in the seat, and they do not support the legs and feet so as to raise the knees, generally a great relief to invalids sitting up. To support the patient's frame, at as many points as possible, is essential. And this is what invalid chairs do *not* do; and when the patient is in, he cannot get out.

IX. LIGHT.

1   It is the unqualified result of all my experience with the sick, that second only to their need of fresh air is their need of light; that, after a close room, what hurts them most is a dark room, and that it is not only light but direct sun-light they want. You had better carry your patient about after the sun, according to the aspect of the rooms, if circumstances permit, than let him linger in a room when the sun is off. People think the effect is upon the spirits only. This is by no means the case. The sun is not only a painter but a sculptor. You admit that he does the photograph. Without going into any scientific exposition, we must admit that light has quite as real and tangible effects upon the human body. But this is not all. Who has not observed the purifying effect of light, and especially of direct sunlight, upon the air of a room? Here is an observation within everybody's experience. Go into a room where the shutters are always shut, (in a sick room or a bedroom there should never be shutters shut), and though the room be uninhabited, though the air has never been polluted by the breathing of human beings, you will observe a close, musty smell of corrupt air, of air, *i.e.* unpurified by the effect of the sun's rays. The mustiness of dark rooms and corners, indeed, is proverbial. The cheerfulness of a room, the usefulness of light in treating disease is all-important.   *Light essential to both health and recovery.*

2   A very high authority in hospital construction has said that people do not enough consider the difference between wards and dormitories   *Aspect, view, and sunlight, matters of first importance to the sick.*

in planning their buildings. But I go farther, and say, that healthy people never remember the difference between *bed-* rooms and *sick-* rooms, in making arrangements for the sick. To a sleeper in health it does not signify what the view is from his bed. He ought never to be in it excepting when asleep, and at night. Aspect does not very much signify either (provided the sun reach his bed-rooms some time in every day, to purify the air), because he ought never to be in his bed-room except during the hours when there is no sun. But the case is exactly reversed with the sick, even should they be as many hours out of their beds as you are in yours, which probably they are not. Therefore, that they should be able, without raising themselves or turning in bed, to see out of a window from their beds, to see sky and sun-light at least, if you can show them nothing else, I assert to be, if not of the very first importance for recovery, at least something very near it. And you should therefore look to the position of the beds of your sick one of the very first things. If they can see out of two windows instead of one, so much the better. Again, the morning sun and the mid-day sun—the hours when they are quite certain not to be up, are of more importance to them, if a choice must be made, than the afternoon sun. Perhaps you can take them out of bed in the afternoon and set them by the window, where they can see the sun. But the best rule is, if possible, to give them direct sun-light from the moment he rises till the moment he sets.

3   Another great difference between the *bed-* room and the *sick-* room is, that the *sleeper* has a very large balance of fresh air to begin with, when he begins the night, if his room has been open all day as it ought to be; the *sick* man has not, because all day he has been breathing the air in the same room, and dirtying it by the emanations from himself. Far more care is therefore necessary to keep up a constant change of air in the sick room.

4   It is hardly necessary to add that there are acute cases, (particularly a few ophthalmic cases, and diseases where the eye is morbidly sensitive), where a subdued light is necessary. But a dark north room is inadmissible even for these. You can always moderate the light by blinds and curtains.

5   Heavy, thick, dark window or bed curtains should, however, hardly ever be used for any kind of sick in this country. A light white curtain at the head of the bed is, in general, all that is necessary,

and a green blind to the window, to be drawn down only when necessary.

6   One of the greatest observers of human things (not physiological), says, in another language, "Where there is sun there is thought." All physiology goes to confirm this. Where is the shady side of deep valleys, there is cretinism. Where are cellars and the unsunned sides of narrow streets, there is the degeneracy and weakliness of the human race—mind and body equally degenerating. Put the pale withering plant and human being into the sun, and, if not too far gone, each will recover health and spirit.

_{Without sunlight we degenerate body and mind.}

7   It is a curious thing to observe how almost all patients lie with their faces turned to the light, exactly as plants always make their way towards the light; a patient will even complain that it gives him pain "lying on that side." "Then why *do* you lie on that side?" He does not know,—but we do. It is because it is the side towards the window. A fashionable physician has recently published in a government report that he always turns his patients' faces from the light. Yes, but nature is stronger than fashionable physicians, and depend upon it she turns the faces back and *towards* such light as she can get. Walk through the wards of a hospital, remember the bed sides of private patients you have seen, and count how many sick you ever saw lying with their faces towards the wall.

_{Almost all patients lie with their faces to the light.}

X. CLEANLINESS OF ROOMS AND WALLS.

1   It cannot be necessary to tell a nurse that she should be clean or that she should keep her patient clean,—seeing that the greater part of nursing consists in preserving cleanliness. No ventilation can freshen a room or ward where the most scrupulous cleanliness is not observed. Unless the wind be blowing through the windows at the rate of twenty miles an hour, dusty carpets, dirty wainscots, musty curtains and furniture, will infallibly produce a close smell. I have lived in a large and expensively furnished London house, where the only constant inmate in two very lofty rooms, with opposite windows, was myself, and yet, owing to the abovementioned dirty circumstances, no opening of windows could ever keep those rooms free from closeness; but the carpet and curtains having been turned out of the rooms altogether, they became instantly as fresh as could be wished. It is pure nonsense to say that in London a room cannot be kept clean. Many of our hospitals show the exact reverse.

Cleanliness of carpets and furniture.

2   But no particle of dust is ever or can ever be removed or really got rid of by the present system of dusting. Dusting in these days means nothing but flapping the dust from one part of a room on to another with doors and windows closed. What you do it for I cannot think. You had much better leave the dust alone, if you are not going to take it away altogether. For from the time a room begins to be a room up to the time when it ceases to be one, no one atom of dust ever actually leaves its precincts. Tidying a room means nothing

Dust never removed now.

now but removing a thing from one place, which it has kept clean for itself, on to another and a dirtier one. Flapping by way of cleaning is only admissible in the case of pictures, or anything made of paper. The only way I know to *remove* dust, the plague of all lovers of fresh air, is to wipe everything with a damp cloth. And all furniture ought to be so made as that it may be wiped with a damp cloth without injury to itself, and so polished as that it may be damped without injury to others. To dust, as it is now practised, truly means to distribute dust more equally over a room.

<small>How a room is *dusted*.</small>

3   If you like to clean your furniture by laying out your clean clothes upon your dirty chairs or sofa, this is one way certainly of doing it. Having witnessed the morning process called "tidying the room," for many years, and with ever increasing astonishment, I can describe what it is. From the chairs, tables, or sofa, upon which the "things" have lain during the night, and which are therefore comparatively clean from dust or blacks, the poor *"things"* having "caught" it, they are removed to other chairs, tables, sofas, upon which you could write your name with your finger in the dust or blacks. The *other* side of the "things" is therefore now evenly dirtied or dusted. The housemaid then flaps every things, or some things, not out of her reach, with a thing called a duster—the dust flies up, then re-settles more equally than it lay before the operation. The room has now been "put to rights."

<small>Floors.</small>

4   As to floors, the only really clean floor I know is the Berlin *lackered* floor, which is wet rubbed and dry rubbed every morning to remove the dust. The French *parquet* is always more or less dusty, although infinitely superior in point of cleanliness and healthiness to our absorbent floor.

5   For a sick room, a carpet is perhaps the worst expedient which could by any possibility have been invented. If you must have a carpet, the only safety is to take it up two or three times a year, instead of once. A dirty carpet literally infects the room. And if you consider the enormous quantity of organic matter from the feet of people coming in, which must saturate it, this is by no means surprising.

<small>Washing floors.</small>

6   Washing floors of sick rooms is most objectionable, for this reason. In any school-room or ward, much inhabited, a smell, while the floor is being scoured, quite different from that of soap and water,

is very perceptible. It is the exhalation from the organic matter which has saturated the absorbing floor from the feet and breath of the inhabitants.

7 This is one cause of erysipelas in hospitals.

8 Dry dirt is comparatively safe dirt. Wet dirt becomes dangerous.

9 Uncleansed towns in dry climates have been made pestilential by having a water-supply.

10 Doctors have proscribed scrubbing in hospitals. And nurses have done it in the earliest morning, so as not to be detected.

11 What is to be done?

12 In the sick room, the doctor should always be asked whether and at what hour he chooses the floor to be washed. If a patient can be moved, it will probably be best to wash the floor only when he can be taken into another room, and his own room dried by fire and opened windows before he returns. A dry day and not a damp one is, therefore, necessary.

13 But a private sick room (where there is not the same going to and fro as in a hospital ward) has been kept perfectly clean by wiping the floor with a damp cloth and drying it with a floor-brush.

14 All the furniture was wiped in the same way with a cloth wrung out of hot water—thus freeing the room from dust.

15 This was in an operation case.

16 In more than one hospital the purpose has been answered by planing the floors, saturating them with "drying" linseed oil, well rubbed in, staining them (for the sake of appearance merely), and using beeswax and turpentine.

17 The floor was cleaned by using a brush with a cloth tied over it. And if anything offensive was spilt, it was washed off immediately with soap and water and the place dried.

18 I hope the day will come in England when absorbent floors will cease to be ever used, whether in school-rooms, lunatic asylums, hospitals, or houses.

19 As for walls, the worst is the papered wall; the next worst is plaster. But the plaster can be redeemed by frequent lime-washing; the paper requires frequent renewing. A glazed paper gets rid of a good deal of the danger. But the ordinary bed-room paper is all that it ought *not* to be. Papered, plastered, oil-painted walls.

20 A person who has accustomed her senses to compare atmospheres Atmosphere in painted and papered rooms quite distinguishable.

88 Cleanliness of Rooms & Walls

proper and improper, for the sick and for children, could tell, blindfold, the difference of the air in old painted and in old papered rooms, *cæteris paribus*. The latter will always be musty, even with all the windows open.

21 The close connection between ventilation and cleanliness is shown in this. An ordinary light paper will last clean much longer if there is an Arnott's ventilator in the chimney than it otherwise would.

22 The best wall now extant is oil paint. From this you can wash the animal exuviæ.*

23 These are what make a room musty.

<small>Best kind of wall for a sick-room.</small>

24 The best wall for a sick-room or ward that could be made is pure white non-absorbent cement or glass, or glazed tiles, if they were made sightly enough.

25 Air can be soiled just like water. If you blow into water you will soil it with the animal matter from your breath. So it is with air. Air is always soiled in a room where walls and carpets are saturated with animal exhalations.

26 Want of cleanliness, then, in rooms and wards, which you have to guard against, may arise in three ways.

<small>Dirty air from without.</small>

27 1. Dirty air coming in from without, soiled by sewer emanations, the evaporation from dirty streets, smoke, bits of unburnt fuel, bits of straw, bits of horse dung.

<small>Best kind of wall for a house.</small>

28 If people would but cover the outside walls of their houses with plain or encaustic tiles, what an incalculable improvement would there be in light, cleanliness, dryness, warmth, and consequently economy. The play of a fire-engine would then effectually wash the outside of a house. This kind of *walling* would stand next to paving in improving the health of towns.

<small>Dirty air from within.</small>

29 2. Dirty air coming from within, from dust, which you often displace, but never remove. And this recalls what ought to be a *sine qua non*. Have as few ledges in your room or ward as possible. And under no pretence have any ledge whatever out of sight. Dust accumulates there, and will never be wiped off. This is a certain way to soil the air. Besides this, the animal exhalations from your inmates saturate your furniture. And if you never clean your furniture

<small>How to keep your wall clean at the expense of your clothes.</small>

(22) * If you like to wipe your dirty door, or some portion of your dirty wall, by hanging up your clean gown or shawl against it on a peg, this is one way certainly, and the most usual way, and generally the only way of cleaning either door or wall in a bed-room.

properly, how can your rooms or wards be any thing but musty? Ventilate as you please, the rooms will never be sweet. Besides this, there is a constant *degradation,* as it is called, taking place from everything except polished or glazed articles— *E.g.,* in colouring certain green papers arsenic is used. Now in the very dust even, which is lying about in rooms hung with this kind of green paper, arsenic has been distinctly detected. You see your dust is anything but harmless; yet you will let such dust lie about your ledges for months, your rooms for ever.

30   Again, the fire fills the room with coal-dust.

31   3. Dirty air coming from the carpet. Above all, take care of the carpets, that the animal dirt left there by the feet of visitors does not stay there. Floors, unless the grain is filled up and polished, are just as bad. The smell, already mentioned, from the floor of a school-room or ward, when any moisture brings out the organic matter by which it is saturated, might alone be enough to warn us of the mischief that is going on.

Dirty air from the carpet.

32   The outer air, then, can only be kept clean by sanitary improvements, and by consuming smoke. The expense in soap, which this single improvement would save, is quite incalculable.

Remedies.

33   The inside air can only be kept clean by excessive care in the ways mentioned above—to rid the walls, carpets, furniture, ledges, &c., of the organic matter and dust—dust consisting greatly of this organic matter—with which they become saturated, and which is what really makes the room musty.

34   Without cleanliness, you cannot have all the effect of ventilation; without ventilation, you can have no thorough cleanliness.

35   Very few people, be they of what class they may, have any idea of the exquisite cleanliness required in the sick-room. For much of what is here said applies less to the hospital than to the private sick-room. The smoky chimney, the dusty furniture, the utensils emptied but once a day, often keep the air of the sick constantly dirty in the best private houses.

36   The well have a curious habit of forgetting that what is to them but a trifling inconvenience, to be patiently "put up" with, is to the sick a source of suffering, delaying recovery, if not actually hastening death. The well are scarcely ever more than eight hours, at most, in the same room. Some change they can always make, if only for a

few minutes. Even during the supposed eight hours, they can change their posture or their position in the room. But the sick man, who never leaves his bed, who cannot change by any movement of his own his air, or his light, or his warmth; who cannot obtain quiet, or get out of the smoke, or the smell, or the dust; he is really poisoned or depressed by what is to you the merest trifle.

37   "What can't be cured must be endured," is the very worst and most dangerous maxim for a nurse which ever was made. Patience and resignation in her are but other words for carelessness or indifference—contemptible, if in regard to herself; culpable, if in regard to her sick.

XI. PERSONAL CLEANLINESS.

¹ In almost all diseases, the function of the skin is, more or less, disordered; and in many most important diseases nature relieves herself almost entirely by the skin. This is particularly the case with children. But the excretion, which comes from the skin, is left there, unless removed by washing or by the clothes. Every nurse should keep this fact constantly in mind,—for, if she allow her sick to remain unwashed, or their clothing to remain on them after being saturated with perspiration or other excretion, she is interfering injuriously with the natural processes of health just as effectually as if she were to give the patient a dose of slow poison by the mouth. Poisoning by the skin is no less certain than poisoning by the mouth —only it is slower in its operation. *Poisoning by the skin.*

² The amount of relief and comfort experienced by sick after the skin has been carefully washed and dried, is one of the commonest observations made at a sick bed. But it must not be forgotten that the comfort and relief so obtained are not all. They are, in fact, nothing more than a sign that the vital powers have been relieved by removing something that was oppressing them. The nurse, therefore, must never put off attending to the personal cleanliness of her patient under the plea that all that is to be gained is a little relief, which can be quite as well given later. *Ventilation and skin-cleanliness equally essential.*

³ In all well-regulated hospitals this ought to be, and generally is, attended to. But it is very generally neglected with private sick.

4   Just as it is necessary to renew the air round a sick person frequently, to carry off morbid effluvia from the lungs and skin, by maintaining free ventilation, so is it necessary to keep the pores of the skin free from all obstructing excretions. The object, both of ventilation and of skin-cleanliness is pretty much the same,—to wit, removing noxious matter from the system as rapidly as possible.

5   Care should be taken in all these operations of sponging, washing, and cleansing the skin, not to expose too great a surface at once, so as to check the perspiration, which would renew the evil in another form.

6   The various ways of washing the sick need not here be specified, —the less so as the doctors ought to say which is to be used.

7   In several forms of diarrhœa, dysentery, &c., where the skin is hard and harsh, the relief afforded by washing with a great deal of soft soap is incalculable. In other cases, sponging with tepid soap and water, then with tepid water and drying with a hot towel will be ordered.

8   Every nurse ought to be careful to wash her hands very frequently during the day. If her face, too, so much the better.

9   One word as to cleanliness merely as cleanliness.

Steaming and rubbing the skin.

10   Compare the dirtiness of the water in which you have washed when it is cold without soap, cold with soap, hot with soap. You will find the first has hardly removed any dirt at all, the second a little more, the third a great deal more. But hold your hand over a cup of hot water for a minute or two, and then, by merely rubbing with the finger, you will bring off flakes of dirt or dirty skin. After a vapour bath you may peel your whole self clean in this way. What I mean is, that by simply washing or sponging with water you do not really clean your skin. Take a rough towel, dip one corner in very hot water,—if a little spirit be added to it it will be more effectual,—and then rub as if you were rubbing the towel into your skin with your finger. The black flakes which will come off will convince you that you were not clean before, however much soap and water you have used. These flakes are what require removing. And you can really keep yourself cleaner with a tumbler of hot water and a rough towel and rubbing, than with a whole apparatus of bath and soap and sponge, without rubbing. It is quite nonsense to say that anybody need be dirty. Patients have been kept as clean by these means on a long voyage, when a

11 Washing, however, with a large quantity of water has quite other effects than those of mere cleanliness. The skin absorbs the water and becomes softer and more perspirable. To wash with soap and soft water is, therefore, desirable from other points of view than that of cleanliness.

12 But the water must be soft. People very little think of this. They think mainly of hard water as chapping their hands, not as being a promoter of drunkenness, uncleanliness, indigestion. It is very little observed that "water-dressings," every day more used by surgeons, have absolutely the opposite effect, viz., poisoning the sore, when made with very hard water, to what they have, viz. cleansing and healing the sore, when the water is soft. When water is hard, it is worth while to have distilled water for every water-dressing. For all washing of the sick, it is worth while to collect rain-water, or condense steam from a boiler, or to boil water, which will often remove from one-half to three-fourths of the hardness. Soap and *hard* water actually dirty your patient's skin. The oil in the soap, the exudations from the skin, and the lime in the water, unite to form a kind of varnish upon the skin, which comes off in the above-mentioned black flakes when rubbed.

Soft water.

13 The use of soft or filtered water for making tea or drinks, boiling vegetables, or mixing medicines, is very important. A careless nurse sometimes takes the water from the wash-hand stand for this last purpose. She had often as well not give the medicine at all.

basin full of water could not be afforded, and when they could not be moved out of their berths, as if all the appurtenances of home had been at hand.

XII. CHATTERING HOPES AND ADVICES.

1   The sick man to his advisers.

2   "My advisers! Their name is Legion. * * * Somehow or other, it seems a provision of the universal destinies, that every man, woman, and child should consider him, her, or itself privileged especially to advise me. Why? That is precisely what I want to know." And this is what I have to say to them. I have been advised to go to every place extant in and out of England—to take every kind of exercise by every kind of cart, carriage—yes, and even swing (!) and dumb-bell (!) in existence; to imbibe every different kind of stimulus that ever has been invented. And this when those *best* fitted to know, viz., medical men, after long and close attendance, had declared any journey out of the question, had prohibited any kind of motion whatever, had closely laid down the diet and drink. What would my advisers say, were they the medical attendants, and I, the patient, left their advice, and took the casual adviser's? But the singularity in Legion's mind is this: it never occurs to him that everybody else is doing the same thing, and that I the patient *must* perforce say, in sheer self-defence, like Rosalind, "I could not do with all."

Advising the sick.

3   "Chattering Hopes" may seem an odd heading. But I really believe there is scarcely a greater worry which invalids have to endure than the incurable hopes of their friends. There is no one practice against which I can speak more strongly from actual personal ex-

Chattering hopes the bane of the sick.

perience, wide and long, of its effects during sickness observed both upon others and upon myself. I would appeal most seriously to all friends, visitors, and attendants of the sick to leave off this practice of attempting to "cheer" the sick by making light of their danger and by exaggerating their probabilities of recovery.

4   Far more now than formerly does the medical attendant tell the truth to the sick who are really desirous to hear it about their own state.

5   How intense is the folly, then, to say the least of it, of the friend, be he even a medical man, who thinks that his opinion, given after a cursory observation, will weigh with the patient, against the opinion of the medical attendant, given, perhaps after years of observation, after using every help to diagnosis afforded by the stethoscope, the examination of pulse, tongue, &c.; and certainly after much more observation than the friend can possibly have had.

6   Supposing the patient to be possessed of common sense,—how can the "favourable" opinion, if it is to be called an opinion at all, of the casual visitor "cheer" him,—when different from that of the experienced attendants. Unquestionably the latter may, and often does, turn out to be wrong. But which is most likely to be wrong?

Patient does not want to talk of himself.

7   The fact is, that the patient* is not "cheered" at all by these well-meaning, most tiresome friends. On the contrary, he is de-

Absurd statistical comparisons made in common conversation by sensible people for the benefit of the sick.

(7)   * There are, of course, cases, as in first confinements, when an assurance from the doctor or experienced nurse to the frightened suffering woman that there is nothing unusual in her case, that she has nothing to fear but a few hours' pain, may cheer her most effectually. This is advice of quite another order. It is the advice of experience to utter inexperience. But the advice we have been referring to is the advice of inexperience to bitter experience; and, in general, amounts to nothing more than this, that you think I shall recover from consumption, because somebody knows somebody somewhere who has recovered from fever.

I have heard a doctor condemned whose patient did not, alas! recover, because another doctor's patient of a different sex, of a different age, recovered from a different disease, in a different place. Yes, this is really true. If people who make these comparisons did but know (only they do not care to know), the care and preciseness with which such comparisons require to be made, (and are made), in order to be of any value whatever, they would spare their tongues. In comparing the deaths of one hospital with those of another, any statistics are justly considered absolutely valueless which do not give the ages, the sexes, and the diseases of all the cases. It does not seem necessary to mention this. It does not seem necessary to say that there can be no comparison between old men with dropsies and young women with consumptions. Yet the cleverest men and the cleverest women are often heard making such comparisons, ignoring entirely sex, age, disease, place—in fact, all the conditions essential to the question. It is the merest gossip.

pressed and wearied. If, on the one hand, he exerts himself to tell each successive member of this too numerous conspiracy, whose name is Legion, why he does not think as they do,—in what respect he is worse,—what symptoms exist that they know nothing of,—he is fatigues instead of "cheered," and his attention is fixed upon himself. In general, patients who are really ill, do not want to talk about themselves. Hypochondriacs do, but again I say we are not on the subject of hypochondriacs.

8   If, on the other hand, and which is much more frequently the case, the patient says nothing, but the Shakesperian "Oh!" "Ah!" "Go to!" and "In good sooth!" in order to escape from the conversation about himself the sooner, he is depressed by want of sympathy. He feels isolated in the midst of friends. He feels what a convenience it would be, if there were any single person to whom he could speak simply and openly, without pulling the string upon himself of this shower-bath of silly hopes and encouragements; to whom he could express his wishes and directions without that person persisting in saying "I hope that it will please God yet to give you twenty years," or, "You have a long life of activity before you." How often we see at the end of biographies, or of cases recorded in medical papers, "after a long illness A. died rather suddenly," or, "unexpectedly, both to himself and to others." "Unexpectedly" to others, perhaps, who did not see, because they did not look; but by no means "unexpectedly to himself," as I feel entitled to believe, both from the internal evidence in such stories, and from watching similar cases: there was every reason to expect that A. would die, and he knew it; but he found it useless to insist upon his knowledge to his friends.

<small>Absurd consolations put forth for the benefit of the sick.</small>

9   In these remarks I am alluding neither to acute cases which terminate rapidly nor to "nervous" cases.

10   By the first much interest in their own danger is very rarely felt. In writings of fiction, whether novels or biographies, these death-beds are generally depicted as almost seraphic in lucidity of intelligence. Sadly large has been my experience in death-beds, and I can only say that I have seldom or never seen such. Indifference, excepting with regard to bodily suffering, or to some duty the dying man desires to perform, is the far more usual state.

11   The "nervous case," on the other hand, delights in figuring to himself and others a fictitious danger.

12   But the long chronic case, who knows too well himself, and who has been told by his physician that he will never enter active life again, who feels that every month he has to give up something he could do the month before—oh! spare such sufferers your chattering hopes. You do not know how you worry and weary them. Such real sufferers cannot bear to talk of themselves, still less to hope for what they cannot at all expect.

13   So also as to all the advice showered so profusely upon such sick, to leave off some occupation, to try some other doctor, some other house, climate, pill, powder, or specific; I say nothing of the inconsistency, for these advisers are sure to be the same persons who exhorted the sick man not to believe his own doctor's prognostics, because "doctors are always mistaken," but to believe some other doctor, because "this doctor is always right." Sure also are these advisers to be the persons to bring the sick man fresh occupation, while exhorting him to leave his own.

Wonderful presumption of the advisers of the sick.

14   Wonderful is the face with which friends, lay and medical, will come in and worry the patient with recommendations to do something or other, having just as little knowledge as to its being feasible, or even safe for him, as if they were to recommend a man to take exercise, not knowing he had broken his leg. What would the friend say, if *he* were the medical attendant, and if the patient because some *other* friend had come in, because somebody, anybody, nobody, had recommended something, anything, nothing, were to disregard *his* orders, and take that other body's recommendation? But people never think of this.

Advisers the same now as two hundred years ago.

15   A celebrated historical personage has related the common-places which, when on the eve of executing a remarkable resolution, were showered in nearly the same words by every one around successively for a period of six months. To these the personage states that it was found least trouble always to reply the same thing, viz., that it could not be supposed that such a resolution had been taken without sufficient previous consideration. To patients enduring every day for years from every friend or acquaintance, either by letter or *vivâ voce,* some torment of this kind, I would suggest the same answer. It would indeed be spared, if such friends and acquaintances would but consider for one moment, that it is probable the patient has heard such advice at least fifty times before, and that, had it been practicable,

it would have been practised long ago. But of such consideration there appears to be no chance. Strange, though true, that people should be just the same in these things as they were a few hundred years ago!

16   To me these commonplaces, leaving their smear upon the cheerful, single-hearted, constant devotion to duty, which is so often seen in the decline of such sufferers, recall the slimy trail left by the snail on the sunny southern garden-wall loaded with fruit.

17   No mockery in the world is so hollow as the advice showered upon the sick. It is of no use for the sick to say anything, for what the adviser wants is, *not* to know the truth about the state of the patient, but to turn whatever the sick may say to the support of his own argument, set forth, it must be repeated, without any inquiry whatever into the patient's real condition. "But it would be impertinent or indecent in me to make such an inquiry," says the adviser. True; and how much more impertinent is it to give your advice when you can know nothing about the truth, and admit you could not inquire into it.

Mockery of the advice given to sick.

18   To nurses I say—these are the visitors who do your patient harm. When you hear him told:—1. That he has nothing the matter with him, and that he wants cheering. 2. That he is committing suicide, and that he wants preventing. 3. That he is the tool of somebody who makes use of him for a purpose. 4. That he will listen to nobody, but is obstinately bent upon his own way; and 5. That he ought to be called to the sense of duty, and is flying in the face of Providence;—then know that your patient is receiving all the injury that he can receive from a visitor.

19   How little the real sufferings of illness are known or understood. How little does any one in good health fancy him or even *her*self into the life of a sick person.

20   Do, you who are about the sick or who visit the sick, try and give them pleasure, remember to tell them what will do so. How often in such visits the sick person has to do the whole conversation, exerting his own imagination and memory, while you would take the visitor, absorbed in his own anxieties, making no effort of memory or imagination, for the sick person. "Oh! my dear, I have so much to think of, I really quite forgot to tell him that; besides, I thought he would know it," says the visitor to another friend. How could "he know it"? Depend upon it, the people who say this are really those who have

Means of giving pleasure to the sick.

little "to think of." There are many burthened with business who always manage to keep a pigeonhole in their minds, full of things to tell the "invalid."

21   I do not say, don't tell him your anxieties—I believe it to be good for him and good for you too; but if you tell him what is anxious, surely you can remember to tell him what is pleasant too.

22   A sick person does so enjoy hearing good news:—for instance, of a love and courtship, while in progress to a good ending. If you tell him only when the marriage takes place, he loses half the pleasure, which God knows he has little enough of; and ten to one but you have told him of some love-making with a bad ending.

23   A sick person also intensely enjoys hearing of any *material* good, any positive or practical success of the right. He has so much of books and fiction, of principles, and precepts, and theories; do, instead of advising him with advice he has heard at least fifty times before, tell him of one benevolent act which has really succeeded practically,—it is like a day's health to him. *

24   You have no idea what the craving of sick with undiminished power of thinking, but little power of doing, is to hear of good practical action, when they can no longer partake in it.

25   Do observe these things, especially with invalids. Do remember how their life is to them disappointed and incomplete. You see them lying there with miserable disappointments, from which they can have no escape but death, and you can't remember to tell them of what would give them so much pleasure, or at least an hour's variety.

26   They don't want you to be lachrymose and whining with them, they like you to be fresh and active and interested, but they cannot bear absence of mind, and they are so tired of the advice and preaching they receive from every body, no matter whom it is, they see.

27   There is no better society than babies and sick people for one another. Of course you must manage this so that neither shall suffer from it, which is perfectly possible. If you think the "air of the sick room" bad for the baby, why it is bad for the invalid too, and, there-

(23)   * A small pet animal is often an excellent companion for the sick, for long chronic cases especially. A bird in a cage is sometimes the only pleasure of an invalid confined for years to the same room. If he can feed and clean the animal himself, he ought always to be encouraged and assisted to do so. An invalid, in giving an account of his nursing by a nurse and a dog, infinitely preferred that of the dog; "above all, it did not talk."

fore, you will of course correct it for both. It freshens up a sick person's whole mental atmosphere to see "the baby." And a very young child, if unspoiled, will generally adapt itself wonderfully to the ways of a sick person, if the time they spend together is not too long.

28   If you knew how unreasonably sick people suffer from reasonable causes of distress, you would take more pains about all these things. An infant laid upon the sick bed will do the sick person, thus suffering, more good than all your eloquence. A piece of good news will do the same. Perhaps you are afraid of "disturbing" him. You say there is no comfort for his present cause of affliction. It is perfectly reasonable. The distinction is this, if he is obliged to act, do not "disturb" him with another subject of thought just yet; help him to do what he wants to do: but, if he *has* done this, or if nothing *can* be done, then "disturb" him by all means. You will relieve, more effectually, unreasonable suffering from reasonable causes by telling him "the news," showing him "the baby," or giving him something new to think of or to look at than by all the logic in the world.

29   It has been very justly said that sick and invalids are like children in this, there is no *proportion* in events to them. Now it is your business as their visitor to restore this right proportion for them—to show them what the rest of the world is doing. How can they find it out otherwise? You will find them far more open to conviction than children in this. And you will find that their unreasonable intensity of suffering from unkindness, from want of sympathy, &c., will disappear with their freshened interest in the big world's events. But then you must be able to give them real interests, not gossip.

Note.—There are two classes of patients which are unfortunately becoming more common every day, especially among women of the richer orders, to whom all these remarks are pre-eminently inapplicable. 1. Those who make health an excuse for doing nothing, and at the same time allege that the being able to do nothing is their only grief. 2. Those who have brought upon themselves ill-health by over pursuit of amusement, which they and their friends have most unhappily called intellectual activity. I scarcely know a greater injury that can be inflicted than the advice too often given to the first class "to vegetate"—or than the admiration too often bestowed on the latter class for "pluck."

Two new classes of patients peculiar to this generation.

XIII. OBSERVATION OF THE SICK.

¹ There is no more silly or universal question scarcely asked than this, "Is he better?" Ask it of the medical attendant, if you please. But of whom else, if you wish for a real answer to your question, would you ask it? Certainly not of the casual visitor; certainly not of the nurse, while the nurse's observation is so little exercised as it is now. What you want are facts, not opinions—for who can have any opinion of any value as to whether the patient is better or worse, excepting the constant medical attendant, or the really observing nurse?

² The most important practical lesson that can be given to nurses is to teach them what to observe—how to observe—what symptoms indicate improvement—what the reverse—which are of importance —which are of none—which are the evidence of neglect—and of what kind of neglect.

³ All this is what ought to make part, and an essential part, of the training of every nurse. At present how few there are, either professional or unprofessional, who really know at all whether any sick person they may be with is better or worse.

⁴ The vagueness and looseness of the information one receives in answer to that much abused question, "Is he better?" would be ludicrous, if it were not painful. The only sensible answer (in the present state of knowledge about sickness) would be "How can I know? I cannot tell how he was when I was not with him."

What is the use of the question, Is he better?

5   I can record but a very few specimens of the answers which I have heard made by friends and nurses, and accepted by physicians and surgeons at the very bed-side of the patient, who could have contradicted every word but did not—sometimes from amiability, often from shyness, oftenest from languor!

6   "How often have the bowels acted, nurse?" "Once, sir." This generally means that the utensil has been emptied once, it having been used perhaps seven or eight times.

7   "Do you think the patient is much weaker than he was six weeks ago?" "Oh no, sir; you know it is very long since he has been up and dressed, and he can get across the room now." This means that the nurse has not observed that whereas six weeks ago he sat up and occupied himself in bed, he now lies still doing nothing; that, although he can "get across the room," he cannot stand for five seconds.

8   Another patient who is eating well, recovering steadily, although slowly, from fever, but cannot walk or stand, is represented to the doctor as making no progress at all.

Want of truth the result of want of observation.

9   It is a much more difficult thing to speak the truth than people commonly imagine. There is the want of observation *simple,* and the want of observation *compound,* compounded, that is, with the imaginative faculty. Both may equally intend to speak the truth. The information of the first is simply defective. That of the second is much more dangerous. The first gives, in answer to a question asked about a thing that has been before his eyes perhaps for years, information exceedingly imperfect, or says, he does not know. He has never observed. And people simply think him stupid.

10   The second has observed just as little, but imagination immediately steps in, and he describes the whole thing from imagination merely, being perfectly convinced all the while that he has seen or heard it; or he will repeat a whole conversation, as if it were information which had been addressed to him; whereas it is merely what he has himself said to somebody else. This is the commonest of all. These people do not even observe that they have *not* observed nor remember that they have forgotten.

11   Courts of justice seem to think that any body can speak "the whole truth and nothing but the truth," if he does but intend it. It requires many faculties combined of observation and memory to speak "the whole truth" and to say "nothing but the truth."

12   "I knows I fibs dreadful: but believe me, Miss, I never finds out I have fibbed until they tells me so," was a remark actually made. It is also one of much more extended application than most people have the least idea of.

13   Concurrence of testimony, which is so often adduced as final proof, may prove nothing more, as is well known to those accustomed to deal with the unobservant imaginative, than that one person has told his story a great many times.

14   I have heard thirteen persons "concur" in declaring that a fourteenth, who had never left his bed, went to a distant chapel every morning at seven o'clock.

15   I have heard persons in perfect good faith declare, that a man came to dine every day at the house where they lived, who had never dined there once; that a person had never taken the sacrament, by whose side they had twice at least knelt at Communion; that but one meal a day come out of a hospital kitchen, which for six weeks they had seen provide from three to five and six meals a day. Such instances might be multiplied *ad infinitum* if necessary.

16   Questions as asked now (but too generally) of, or about patients, would obtain no information at all about them, even if the person asked of had every information to give. The question is generally a leading question: and it is singular that people never think what must be the answer to this question before they ask it: for instance, "Has he had a good night?" Now, one patient will think he has a bad night if he has not slept ten hours without waking. Another does not think he has a bad night if he has had intervals of dosing occasionally. The same answer has actually been given as regarded two patients—one who had been entirely sleepless for five times twenty-four hours, and died of it, and another who had not slept the sleep of a regular night, without waking. Why cannot the question be asked, How many hours' sleep has —— had? and at what hours of the night? This is important, because on this depends what the remedy will be. If a patient sleeps two or three hours early in the night, and then does not sleep again at all, ten to one it is not a narcotic he wants, but food or stimulus, or perhaps only warmth. If on the other hand, he is restless and awake all night, and is drowsy in the morning, he probably wants sedatives, either quiet, coolness, or medicine, a lighter diet, or all four. Now the doctor should be told this, or how can he judge what

Leading questions useless or misleading.

106 Observation of The Sick

to give? "I have never closed my eyes all night," an answer as frequently made when the speaker has had several hours' sleep as when he has had none, would then be less often said. Lies, intentional and unintentional, are much seldomer told in answer to precise than to leading questions. Another frequent error is to inquire, whether one cause remains, and not whether the effect which may be produced by a great many different causes, *not* inquired after, remains. As when it is asked, whether there was noise in the street last night; and if there were not, the patient is reported, without more ado, to have had a good night. Patients are completely taken aback by these kinds of leading questions, and give only the exact amount of information asked for, even when they know it to be completely misleading. The shyness of patients is seldom allowed for.

17   How few there are who, by five or six pointed questions, can elicit the whole case and get accurately to know and to be able to report *where* the patient is.

<small>Means of obtaining inaccurate information.</small>

18   I knew a very clever physician, of large dispensary and hospital practice, who invariably began his examination of each patient with "Put your finger where you *be* bad." That man would never waste his time with collecting inaccurate information from nurse or patient. Leading questions always collect inaccurate information.

19   At a recent celebrated trial, the following leading question was put successively to nine distinguished medical men. "Can you attribute these symptoms to anything else but poison?" And out of the nine, eight answered "No!" without any qualification whatever. It appeared, upon cross-examination:—1. That none of them had ever seen a case of the kind of poisoning supposed. 2. That none of them had ever seen a case of the kind of disease to which the death, if not to poison, was attributable. 3. That none of them were even aware of the main fact of the disease and condition to which the death was attributable.

20   Surely nothing stronger can be adduced to prove what use leading questions are of, and what they lead to.

21   I had rather not say how many instances I have known, where, owing to this system of leading questions, the patient has died, and the attendants have been actually unaware of the principal feature of the case.

<small>As to food patient takes or does not take.</small>

22   It is useless to go through all the particulars, besides sleep, in

which people have a peculiar talent for gleaning inaccurate information. As to food, for instance, I often think that most common question, How is your appetite ? can only be put because the questioner believes the questioned has really nothing the matter with him, which is very often the case. But where there is, the remark holds good which has been made about sleep. The *same* answer will often be made as regards a patient who cannot take two ounces of solid food per diem, and a patient who does not enjoy five meals a day as much as usual.

23   Again, the question, How is your appetite? is often put when How is your digestion? is the question meant. No doubt the two things often depend on one another. But they are quite different. Many a patient can eat, if you can only "tempt his appetite." The fault lies in your not having got him the thing that he fancies. But many another patient does not care between grapes and turnips,—everything is equally distasteful to him. He would try to eat anything which would do him good; but everything "makes him worse." The fault here generally lies in the cooking. It is not his "appetite" which requires "tempting," it is his digestion which requires sparing. And good sick cookery will save the digestion half its work.

24   There may be four different causes, any one of which will produce the same result, viz., the patient slowly starving to death from want of nutrition.
   1. Defect in cooking;
   2. Defect in choice of diet;
   3. Defect in choice of hours for taking diet;
   4. Defect of appetite in patient.
Yet all these are generally comprehended in the one sweeping assertion that the patient has "no appetite."

25   Surely many lives might be saved by drawing a closer distinction; for the remedies are as diverse as the causes. The remedy for the first is, to cook better; for the second, to choose other articles of diet; for the third, to watch for the hours when the patient is in want of food; for the fourth, to show him what he likes, and sometimes unexpectedly. But no one of these remedies will do for any other of the defects not corresponding with it.

26   It cannot too often be repeated that patients are generally either too languid to observe these things, or too shy to speak about them;

108 Observation of The Sick

nor is it well that they should be made to observe them, it fixes their attention upon themselves.

27   Again, I say, what *is* the nurse or friend there for except to take note of these things, instead of the patient doing so?

<small>More important to spare the patient thought than physical exertion.</small>

28   It is commonly supposed that the nurse is there to spare the patient from making physical exertion for himself—I would rather say, that she ought to be there to spare him from taking thought for himself. And I am quite sure, that if the patient were spared all thought for himself and *not* spared all physical exertion, he would be the gainer. The reverse is generally the case in the private house. In the hospital it is the relief from all anxiety, afforded by the rules of a well-regulated institution, which has often such a beneficial effect upon the patient.

29   "Can I do anything for you?" says the thoughtless nurse—and the uncivil patient invariably answers "no"—the civil patient, "no thank you." The fact is, that a real patient will rather go without almost anything than make the exertion of thinking *what* the nurse has left undone. And surely it is for her, not for him, to make this exertion. Such a question is, on her part, a mere piece of laziness, under the guise of being "obliging." She wishes to throw the trouble on the patient of nursing himself.

<small>Means of obtaining inaccurate information as to diarrhœa.</small>

30   Again, the question is sometimes put, Is there diarrhœa? And the answer will be the same, whether it is just merging into cholera, whether it is a trifling degree brought on by some trifling indiscretion, which will cease the moment the cause is removed, or whether there is no diarrhœa at all, but simply relaxed bowels.

31   It is useless to multiply instances of this kind. As long as observation is so little cultivated as it is now, I do believe that it is better for the physician *not* to see the friends of the patient at all. They will oftener mislead him than not. And as often by making the patient out worse as better than he really is.

32   In the case of infants, *everything* must depend upon the accurate observation of the nurse or mother who has to report. And how seldom is this condition of accuracy fulfilled.

33   It is the real test of a nurse whether she can nurse a sick infant. Of *it* she can never ask, Can I do anything for you?

<small>Means of cultivating sound and ready observation.</small>

34   A celebrated man, though celebrated only for foolish things, has told us that one of his main objects in the education of his son, was

to give him a ready habit of accurate observation, a certainty of perception, and that for this purpose one of his means was a month's course as follows:—he took the boy rapidly past a toy-shop; the father and son then described to each other as many of the objects as they could, which they had seen in passing the windows, noting them down with pencil and paper, and returning afterwards to verify their own accuracy. The boy always succeeded best, *e.g.,* if the father described 30 objects, the boy did 40, and scarcely ever made a mistake.

35   How wise a piece of education this would be for much higher objects; and in our calling of nurses the thing itself is essential. For it may safely be said, not that the habit of ready and correct observation will by itself make us useful nurses, but that without it we shall be useless with all our devotion.

36   One nurse in charge of a set of wards not only carries in her head all the little varieties in the diets which each patient is allowed to fix for himself, but also exactly what each patient has taken during each day. Another nurse, in charge of one single patient, takes away his meals day after day all but untouched, and never knows it.

37   If you find it helps you to note down such things on a bit of paper, in pencil, by all means do so. Perhaps it more often lames than strengthens the memory and observation. But if you cannot get the habit of observation one way or other, you had better give up the being a nurse, for it is not your calling, however kind and anxious you may be.

38   Surely you can learn at least to judge with the eye how much an oz. of solid food is, how much an oz. of liquid. You will find this helps your observation and memory very much, you will then say to yourself "A. took about an oz. of his meat to day;" "B. took three times in 24 hours about $\frac{1}{4}$ pint of beef tea;" instead of saying "B. has taken nothing all day," or "I gave A. his dinner as usual."

39   I have known several of our real old-fashioned hospital "sisters," who could, as accurately as a measuring glass, measure out all their patient's wine and medicine by the eye, and never be wrong. I do not recommend this,—one must be very sure of one's self to do it. I only mention it, because if a nurse can by practice measure medicine by the eye, surely she is no nurse who cannot measure by the eye about how much food (in oz.) her patient has taken. In hospitals those who cut up the diets give with quite sufficient accuracy, to each pa-

Sound and ready observation essential in a nurse.

tient, his 12 oz. or his 6 oz. of meat without weighing. Yet a nurse will often have patients loathing all food and incapable of any will to get well, who just tumble over the contents of the plate or dip the spoon in the cup to deceive the nurse, and she will take it away without ever seeing that there is just the same quantity of food as when she brought it, and she will tell the doctor, too, that the patient has eaten all his diets as usual, when all she ought to have meant is that she has taken away his diets as usual.

40 Now what kind of a nurse is this?

English women have great capacity of but little practice in close observation.

41 It may be too broad an assertion, and it certainly sounds like a paradox. But I think that in no country are women to be found so deficient in ready and sound observation as in England, while peculiarly capable of being trained to it. The French or Irish woman is too quick of perception to be so sound an observer—the Teuton is too slow to be so ready an observer as the English woman might be. Yet English women lay themselves open to the charge so often made against them by men, viz., that they are not to be trusted in handicrafts to which their strength is quite equal, for want of a practiced and steady observation. In countries, both Protestant and Roman Catholic, where women, both "secular" and "religious," (with average intelligence certainly not superior to that of, English women) are employed *e.g.*, in dispensing, men responsible for what these women do (not theorizing about man's and woman's "missions"), have stated that they preferred the service of women to that of men, as being more exact, more careful, and incurring fewer mistakes of inadvertence.

42 Now certainly Englishwomen are peculiarly capable of attaining to this.

43 I remember when a child, hearing the story of an accident, related by some one who sent two nieces to fetch a "bottle of salvolatile from her room;" "Mary could not stir," she said, "Fanny ran and fetched a bottle that was not salvolatile, and that was not in my room."

44 Now this habit of inattention generally pursues a person through life. A woman is asked to fetch a large new bound red book, lying on the table by the window, and she fetches five small old boarded brown books lying on the shelf by the fire. And this, though she has "put that room to rights" every day for a month perhaps, and must have observed the books every day, lying in the same places, for a month, if she had any observation.

45   Habitual observation is the more necessary, when any sudden call arises. If "Fanny" had observed "the bottle of salvolatile" in " the aunt's room," every day she was there, she would more probably have found it when it was suddenly wanted.

46   There are two causes for these mistakes of inadvertence, 1. A want of ready attention; only part of the request is heard at all. 2. A want of the habit of observation.

47   To a nurse I would add, take care that you always put the same things in the same places; you don't know how suddenly you may be called on some day to find something, and may not be able to remember in your haste where you yourself had put it, if your memory is not in the habit of seeing the thing there always.

48   Some few of the instances in which nurses frequently fail in observation, may here be mentioned. There is a well-marked distinction between the excitable and what I will call the *accumulative* temperament in patients. One will blaze up at once, under any shock or anxiety, and sleep very comfortably after it; another will seem quite calm and even torpid, under the same shock, and people say, "He hardly felt it at all," yet you will find him some time after slowly sinking. The same remark applies to the action of narcotics, of aperients, which, in the one, take effect directly, in the other not perhaps for twenty-four hours. A journey, a visit, an unwonted exertion, will affect the one immediately, but he recovers after it; the other bears it very well at the time, apparently, and dies or is prostrated for life by it. People often say how difficult the excitable temperament is to manage—I say how difficult is the *accumulative* temperament. With the first you have an out-break which you could anticipate, and it is all over. With the second you never know where you are—you never know when the consequences are over. And it requires your closest observation to know what *are* the consequences of what—for the consequent by no means follows immediately upon the antecedent—and coarse observation is utterly at fault.

Difference of excitable and accumulative temperaments.

49   Almost all superstitions are owing to defective knowledge, to bad observation, to the *post hoc,* *ergo propter hoc;* and bad observers are almost all superstitious. Farmers used to attribute disease among cattle to witchcraft; weddings have been attributed to seeing one magpie, deaths to seeing three; and I have heard the most highly educated now-a-days draw consequences for the sick closely resembling these.

Superstition the fruit of bad observation.

112 Observation of The Sick

<small>Physiognomy of disease little known.</small>

50   Another remark: although there is unquestionably a physiognomy of disease as well as of health; of all parts of the body, the face is perhaps the one which tells the least to the common observer or the casual visitor. Because, of all parts of the body, it is the one most exposed to other influences, besides health. And people never, or scarcely ever, observe enough to know how to distinguish between the effect of exposure, of robust health, of a tender skin of a tendency to congestion, of suffusion, flushing, or many other things. Again, the face is often the last to shew emaciation. I should say that the hand was a much surer test than the face, both as to flesh, colour, ciculation, &c., &c. It is true that there are *some* diseases which are only betrayed at all by something in the face, *e.g.*, the eye or the tongue, as great irritability of brain by the appearance of the pupil of the eye. But we are talking of casual, not minute, observation. And few minute observers will hesitate to say that far more untruth than truth is conveyed by the oft repeated words, He *looks* well, or ill, or better or worse.

51   Wonderful is the way in which people will go upon the slightest observation, or often upon no observation at all, or upon some *saw* which the world's experience, if it had any, would have pronounced utterly false long ago.

52   I have known patients dying of sheer pain, exhaustion, and want of sleep, from one of the most lingering and painful diseases known, preserve, till within a few days of death, not only the healthy colour of the cheek, but the mottled appearance of a robust child. And scores of times have I heard these unfortunate creatures assailed with, "I am glad to see you looking so well." "I see no reason why you should not live till ninety years of age." "Why don't you take a little more exercise and amusement?" with all the other common-places with which we are so familiar.

53   There is, unquestionably, a physiognomy of disease. Let the nurse learn it.

54   The experienced nurse can always tell that a person has taken a narcotic the night before by the patchiness of the colour about the face, when the re-action of depression has set in; that very colour which the inexperienced will point to as a proof of health.

55   There is, again, a faintness, which does not betray itself by the colour at all, or in which the patient becomes brown instead of white.

There is a faintness of another kind which, it is true, can always be seen by the paleness.

56 But the nurse seldom distinguishes. She will talk to the patient who is too faint to move, without the least scruple, unless he is pale and unless, luckily for him, the muscles of the throat are affected and he loses his voice.

57 Yet these two faintnesses are perfectly distinguishable, by the mere countenance of the patient.

58 Again, the nurse must distinguish between the idiosyncracies of patients. One likes to suffer out all his suffering alone, to be as little looked after as possible. Another likes to be perpetually made much of and pitied, and to have some one always by him. Both these peculiarities might be observed and indulged much more than they are. For quite as often does it happen that a busy attendance is forced upon the first patient, who wishes for nothing but to be "let alone," as that the second is left to think himself neglected.

Peculiarities of patients.

59 People have two ways of considering nursing. One is to consider it a troublesome and useless infliction (which it too often is), and to have as little of it as possible. The other is to consider it a "mystery." When a really good nurse is seen inducing a patient to do willingly what another nurse has entirely failed in, people look upon it as "genius," or as a kind of biological trick, such as used to be practised some years ago in London.

60 Now, there is no "mystery" at all about it. Good nursing consists simply in observing the little things which are common to all sick, and those which are particular to each sick individual.

61 Some people have a curious power over animals. They can collect wild birds round them in a wood. This, once thought witchcraft, is now supposed to be some peculiar power, which we can't see into, like the calculating boy's. It is nothing at all but the minute observation of the habits and instincts of birds.

62 So the "peculiar power" of one nurse, and the want of power of another over her patient, is nothing at all but minute observation in the former of what affects him, and want of observation in the latter.

63 In nothing is this more remarkable than in inducing patients to take food. A patient is sinking for want of it under one nurse; you put him under another, and he takes it directly. How is this? People say, oh! she has a command over her patients. It is no command. It is the

114 Observation of The Sick

way she feeds him, or the way she pillows his head, so that he can swallow comfortably. Opening the window will enable one patient to take his food; washing his face and hands another; merely passing a wet towel over the back of the neck, a third; a fourth, who is a depressed suicide, requires a little cheering to give him spirit to eat. The nurse amuses him with giving some variety to his ideas. I remember that, when very ill, the way in which one nurse put the spoon into my mouth enabled me to swallow when I could not if I was fed by any one else.

64   It is just the observation of all these little things, no unintelligible "influence," which enables one woman to save life; it is the want of such observation which prevents another from finding the means to do so.

65   Even delirium, which seems to place the patient so out of the reach of all human relief, that he is shrieking and calling for you and you cannot make him understand that you are there by him, is often increased by an awkward noise or touch, and yet the nurse who does so never perceives it.

Nurse must observe for herself increase of patient's weakness, patient will not tell her.

66   Again, few things press so heavily on one suffering from long and incurable illness, as the necessity of recording in words from time to time, for the information of the nurse, who will not otherwise see, that he cannot do this or that, which he could do a month or a year ago. What is a nurse there for if she cannot observe these things for herself? Yet I have known—and known too among those—and *chiefly* among those—whom money and position put in possession of everything which money and position could give—I have known, I say, more accidents, (fatal, slowly or rapidly,) arising from this want of observation among nurses than from almost anything else. Because a patient could get out of a warm-bath alone a month ago—because a patient could walk as far as his bell a week ago, the nurse concludes that he can do so now. She has never observed the change; and the patient is lost from being left in a helpless state of exhaustion, till some one accidentally comes in. And this not from any unexpected apoplectic, paralytic, or fainting fit (though even these could be expected far more, at least, than they are now, if we did but *observe*). No, from the expected, or to be expected, inevitable, visible, calculable, uninterrupted increase of weakness, which none need fail to observe.

67 Again, a patient not usually confined to bed, is compelled by an attack of diarrhœa, vomiting, or other accident, to keep his bed for a few days; he gets up for the first time, and the nurse lets him go into another room, without coming in, a few minutes afterwards, to look after him. It never occurs to her that he is quite certain to be faint, or cold, or to want something. She says, as her excuse, Oh, he does not like to be fidgetted after. Yes, he said so some weeks ago; but he never said he did not like to be "fidgetted after," when he is in the state he is in now; and if he did, you ought to make some excuse to go in to him. More patients have been lost in this way than is at all generally known, viz., from relapses brought on by being left for an hour or two faint, or cold, or hungry, after getting up for the first time.
Accidents arising from the nurse's want of observation.

68 You do not know how small is the power of resistance in a weak patient—how he will succumb to habits of the nurse, which occasion him positive pain for the time and total prostration for the whole day, rather than remonstrate. A good nurse gets the patient into a good habit, such as washing and dressing at different times so as to spare his strength. A bad nurse succeeds, and the patient adopts her bad ways without a struggle. *Patients do what they are expected to do.* This is equally important to be remembered, for good as well as for bad.

69 Yet it appears that scarcely any improvement in the faculty of observing is being made. Vast has been the increase of knowledge in pathology—that science which teaches us the final change produced by disease on the human frame—scarce any in the art of observing the signs of the change while in progress. Or, rather, is it not to be feared that observation, as an essential part of medicine, has been declining?
Is the faculty of observing on the decline?

70 A high medical authority abroad (in a country where pathology is considered to be even farther advanced than in ours) says, Have you detected anything with the stethoscope? then it is already too late to do any good.

71 Which of us has not heard fifty times, from one or another, a nurse, or a friend of the sick, aye, and a medical friend too, the following remark:—"So A. is worse, or B is dead. I saw him the day before; I thought him so much better; there certainly was no appearance from which one could have expected so sudden (?) a change."

116 Observation of The Sick

I have never heard any one say, though one would think it the more natural thing, "There *must* have been *some* appearance, which I should have seen if I had but looked; let me try and remember what there was, that I may observe another time." No, this is not what people say. They boldly assert that there was nothing to observe, not that their observation was at fault.

72 Let people who have to observe sickness and death look back and try to register in their observation the appearances which have preceded relapse, attack, or death, and not assert that there were none, or that there were not the *right* ones.

<small>Approach of death, paleness by no means an invariable effect, as we find in novels.</small>

73 It falls to few ever to have had the opportunity of observing the different aspects which the human face puts on at the sudden approach of certain forms of death by violence; and as it is a knowledge of little use I only mention it here as being the most startling example of what I mean. In the nervous temperament the face becomes pale (this is the only *recognized* effect); in the sanguine temperament purple; in the bilious yellow, or every manner of colour in patches. Now, it is generally supposed that paleness is the one indication of almost any violent change in the human being, whether from terror, disease, or anything else. There can be no more false observation. Granted, it is the one recognized livery, as I have said— *de rigueur* in novels, but nowhere else.

<small>Observation of general conditions.</small>

74 There are two habits of mind often equally misleading from correct conclusions:—(1.) a want of observation of conditions, and (2.) an inveterate habit of taking averages.

75 1. Men whose profession like that of medical men leads them to observe only, or chiefly, palpable and permanent organic changes are often just as wrong in their opinion of the result as those who do not observe at all. For instance, there is a cancer or a broken leg; the surgeon has only to look at it once to know; it will not be different if he sees it in the morning to what it would have been had he seen it in the evening. In whatever conditions the broken leg is, or is likely to be, there will still be the broken leg, until it is united. The same with many organic diseases. An experienced physician has but to feel the pulse once, and he knows that there is aneurism which will kill some time or other.

76 But with the great majority of cases, there is nothing of the kind; and the power of forming any correct opinion as to the result must

entirely depend upon an enquiry into all the conditions in which the patient lives. In a complicated state of society in large towns, death, as every one of great experience knows, is far less often produced by any one organic disease than by some illness, after many other diseases, producing just the sum of exhaustion necessary for death.

77   There is nothing so absurd, nothing so misleading as the verdict one so often hears: So-and-so has no organic disease,—there is no reason why he should not live to extreme old age; sometimes the clause is added, sometimes not: Provided he has quiet, good food, good air, &c., &c., &c.,; the verdict is repeated by ignorant people *without* the latter clause; or there is no possibility of the conditions of the latter clause being obtained; and this, the *only* essential part of the whole, is made of no effect.

78   I have known two cases, the one of a man who intentionally and repeatedly displaced a dislocation, and was kept and petted by all the surgeons, the other of one who was pronounced to have nothing the matter with him, there being no organic change perceptible, but who died within the week. In both these cases, it was the nurse who, by accurately pointing out what she had accurately observed, to the doctors, saved the one case from persevering in a fraud, the other from being discharged when actually in a dying state.

_{Observes look too much to what is palpable to their senses, not to what is implied by conditions.}

79   But one may even go further and say, that in diseases which have their origin in the feeble or irregular action of some function, and not in organic change, it is quite an accident if the doctor who sees the case only once a day, and generally at the same time, can form any but a negative idea of its real condition. In the middle of the day, when such a patient has been refreshed by light and air, by his tea, his beef tea, and his brandy, by hot bottles to his feet, by being washed and by clean linen, you can scarcely believe that he is the same person as he lay with a rapid fluttering pulse, with puffed eye-lids, with short breath, cold limbs, and unsteady hands, this morning. Now what is a nurse to do in such a case? Not cry, "Lord bless you, sir, why you'd have thought he were a dying all night." This may be true, but it is not the way to impress with the truth a doctor, more capable of forming a judgment from the facts, if he did but know them, than you are. What he wants is not your opinion, however respectfully given, but your facts. In all diseases it is important, but in diseases which do not run a distinct and fixed course, it is not only important,

118 Observation of The Sick

it is essential that the facts the nurse alone can observe, should be accurately observed, and accurately reported to the doctor.

Pulses.

80   The nurse's attention should be directed to the extreme variation there is not unfrequently in the pulse of such patients during the day. A very common case is this: Between 3 and 4 a.m. the pulse becomes quick, perhaps 130, and so thready it is not like a pulse at all, but like a string vibrating just underneath the skin. After this the patient gets no more sleep. About mid-day the pulse has come down to 80; and though feeble and compressible is a very respectable pulse. At night, if the patient has had a day of excitement, it is almost imperceptible. But, if the patient has had a good day, it is stronger and steadier and not quicker than at mid-day. This is a common history of a common pulse; and others, equally varying during the day, might be given. Now, in inflammation, which may almost always be detected by the pulse, in typhoid fever, which is accompanied by the low pulse that nothing will raise, there is no such great variation. And doctors and nurses become accustomed not to look for it. The doctor indeed cannot. But the variation is in itself an important feature.

81   Cases like the above often "go off rather suddenly," as it is called, from some trifling ailment of a few days, which just makes up the sum of exhaustion necessary to produce death. And everybody cries, Who would have thought it? except the observing nurse, if there is one, who had always expected the exhaustion to come, from which there would be no rally, because she knew the patient had no capital in strength on which to draw, if he failed for a few days to make his barely daily income in sleep and nutrition.

82   Really good nurses are often distressed, because they cannot impress the doctor with the real danger of their patient; and quite provoked because the patient "will look," either "so much better" or "so much worse" than he really is "when the doctor is there." The distress is very legitimate, but it generally arises from the nurse not having the power of laying clearly and shortly before the doctor the facts from which she derives her opinion, or from the doctor being hasty and inexperienced, and not capable of eliciting them. A man who really cares for his patients, will soon learn to ask for and appreciate the information of a nurse, who is at once a careful observer and a clear reporter.

83   A nurse ought to be able to understand what the variations of the

pulse imply, what its character indicates. It is not the absolute rate of the pulse which it signifies so much for you to know. At least, you ought to be able to form an accurate enough guess at its rate without counting. It is the character of the pulse which signifies. There is the "splashing" pulse, which implies aneurism. There is the pulse without an edge, which feels not like a ribbon, but a thread running along a space which it does not fill. There is the intermittent pulse of heart disease, the pulse of acute pleurisy, the pulse of peritonitis, the throbbing pulse which indicates acute inflammation or risk of hæmorrhage. There is the rapid pulse of exhaustion in fever, which is the sign that the time has come for wine and stimulants. And upon the seizing of this time the patient's life constantly depends. The administration of the wine brings down the pulse. The doctor leaves orders that if re-action follows on depression, the wine is to be discontinued or the quantity diminished. This re-action is indicated by the pulse.

84 How can the nurse have any confidence in her own work, how can she be the means of saving risk and suffering to her patient, if she is not made familiar with all these characters of pulse?

85 There is the low pulse which indicates the danger of gangrene or pyæmia. There is the pulse of apoplexy, which indicates the danger of bleeding, sometimes practised even by unprofessional persons. There is the pulse of brain disease, the pulse of congestion, and many others. It is impossible to describe them on paper. They must be felt to be known. And it is a knowledge absolutely essential to a real nurse.

86 For this reason it is so necessary that her senses should be cultivated and acute. The same nurse who cannot distinguish by the ear the sound of her patient's bell will certainly not be able to distinguish by the touch the character of his pulse. And she may commit frightful mistakes, which would make it better that she never should have had it put into her head to feel pulses at all.

87 To return to the observation of conditions.

88 I have heard a physician, deservedly eminent, assure the friends of a patient of his recovery. Why? Because he had now prescribed a course, every detail of which the patient had followed for years. And because he had forbidden a course which the patient could not by any possibility alter.

To arrive at a sound judgment not only what the patient is but what he is likely to do must be taken into account.

89 Undoubtedly a person of no scientific knowledge whatever but of observation and experience in these kinds of conditions, will be able to arrive at a much truer guess as to the probable duration of life of members of a family or inmates of a house, than the most scientific physician to whom the same persons are brought to have their pulse felt; no enquiry being made into their conditions.

90 In Life Insurance and such like societies, were they instead of having the persons examined by a medical man, to have the houses, conditions, ways of life, of these persons examined, at how much truer results would they arrive! W. Smith appears a fine hale man, but it might be known that the next cholera epidemic he runs a bad chance. Mr. and Mrs. J. are a strong healthy couple, but it might be known that they live in such a house, in such a part of London, so near the river that they will kill four-fifths of their children; which of the children will be the ones to survive might also be known.

"Average rate of mortality" tells us only that so many per cent. will die. Observation must tell us *which* in the hundred they will be who will die.

91 2. Averages again seduce us away from minute Observation. "Average mortalities" merely tell that so many per cent. die in this town and so many in that, per annum. But whether A. or B. will be among these, the "average rate" of course does not tell. We know, say, that from 22 to 24 per 1,000 will die in London next year. But minute enquiries into conditions enable us to know that in such a district, nay, in such a street,—or even on one side of that street, in such a particular house, or even on one floor of that particular house, will be the excess of mortality, that is, the person will die who ought not to have died before old age.

92 Now, would it not very materially alter the opinion of whoever were endeavouring to form one, if he knew that from that floor of that house of that street the man came?

93 Much more precise might be our observations even than this and much more correct our conclusions.

94 It is well known that the same names may be seen constantly recurring on workhouse books for generations. That is, the persons were born and brought up, and will be born and brought up, generation after generation, in the conditions which make paupers. Death and disease are like the workhouse, they take from the same family, the same house, or in other words the same conditions. Why will we not observe what they are?

95 The close observer may safely predict that such a family, whether

its members marry or not, will become extinct; that such another will degenerate morally and physically. But who learns the lesson? On the contrary, it may be well known that the children die in such a house at the rate of 8 out of 10; one would think that nothing more need be said; for how could Providence speak more distinctly? yet nobody listens, the family goes on living there till it dies out, and then some other family takes it. Neither would they listen "if one rose from the dead."

96   In dwelling upon the vital importance of *sound* observation, it must never be lost sight of what observation is for. It is not for the sake of piling up miscellaneous information or curious facts, but for the sake of saving life and increasing health and comfort. The caution may seem useless, but it is quite surprising how many men (some women do it too), practically behave as if the scientific end were the only one in view, or as if the sick body were but a reservoir for stowing medicines into, and the surgical disease only a curious case the sufferer has made for the attendant's special information. This is really no exaggeration. You think, if you suspected your patient was being poisoned, say, by a copper kettle, you would instantly, as you ought, cut off all possible connection between him and the suspected source of injury, without regard to the fact that a curious mine of observation is thereby lost. But it is not everybody who does so, and it has actually been made a question of medical ethics, what should the medical man do if he suspected poisoning? The answer seems a very simple one,—insist on a confidential nurse being placed with the patient, or give up the case. *What observation is for.*

97   And remember every nurse should be one who is to be depended upon, in other words, capable of being a "confidential" nurse. She does not know how soon she may find herself placed in such a situation; she must be no gossip, no vain talker; she should never answer questions about her sick except to those who have a right to ask them; she must, I need not say, be strictly sober and honest; but more than this, she must be a religious and devoted woman; she must have a respect for her own calling, because God's precious gift of life is often literally placed in her hands; she must be a sound, and close, and quick observer; and she must be a woman of delicate and decent feeling. *What a confidential nurse should be.*

98   To return to the question of what observation is for:—It would *Observation is for practical purposes.*

really seem as if some had considered it as its own end, as if detection, not cure, was their business; nay more, in a recent celebrated trial, three medical men, according to their own account, suspected poison, prescribed for dysentery, and left the patient to the poisoner. This is an extreme case. But in a small way, the same manner of acting falls under the cognizance of us all. How often the attendants of a case have admitted that they knew perfectly well that the patient could not get well in such an air, in such a room, or under such circumstances, yet have gone on dosing him with medicine, and making no effort to remove the poison from him, or him from the poison which they knew was killing him; nay, more, have sometimes not so much as mentioned their conviction in the right quarter—that is, to the only person who could act in the matter.

CONCLUSION.

¹ The whole of the preceding remarks apply even more to children and to puerperal women than to patients in general. They also apply to the nursing of surgical, quite as much as to that of medical cases. Indeed, if it be possible, cases of external injury require such care even more than sick. In surgical wards, one duty of every nurse certainly is *prevention*. Fever, or hospital gangrene, or pyæmia, or purulent discharge of some kind may else supervene. Has she a case of compound fracture, of amputation, or of erysipelas, it may depend very much on how she looks upon the things enumerated in these notes, whether one or other of these hospital diseases attacks her patient or not. If she allows her ward to become filled with the peculiar close fœtid smell, so apt to be produced among surgical cases, especially where there is great suppuration and discharge, she may see a vigorous patient in the prime of life gradually sink and die where, according to all human probability, he ought to have recovered. The surgical nurse must be ever on the watch, ever on her guard, against want of cleanliness, foul air, want of light, and of warmth.

² Nevertheless let no one think that because *sanitary* nursing is the subject of these notes, therefore, what may be called the handicraft of nursing is to be undervalued. A patient may be left to bleed to death in a sanitary palace. Another who cannot move himself may die of bedsores, because the nurse does not know how to change and clean him, while he has every requisite of air, light, and quiet. But

— margin: Sanitary nursing as essential in surgical as in medical cases, but not to supersede surgical nursing.

124 Conclusion

nursing, as a handicraft, has not been treated of here for three reasons: 1. that these notes do not pretend to be a manual for nursing, any more than for cooking for the sick; 2. that the writer, who has herself seen more of what may be called surgical nursing, *i.e.* practical manual nursing, than, perhaps, any one in Europe, honestly believes that it is impossible to learn it from any book, and that it can only be thoroughly learnt in the wards of a hospital; and she also honestly believes that the perfection of surgical nursing may be seen practised by the old-fashioned "Sister" of a London hospital, as it can be seen nowhere else in Europe. 3. While thousands die of foul air, &c., who have this surgical nursing to perfection, the converse is comparatively rare.

Children: their greater susceptibility to the same things.

3   To revert to children. They are much more susceptible than grown people to all noxious influences. They are affected by the same things, but much more quickly and seriously, viz., by want of fresh air, of proper warmth, want of cleanliness in house, clothes, bedding, or body, by startling noises, improper food, or want of punctuality, by dulness and by want of light, by too much or too little covering in bed, or when up,—by want of the spirit of management generally in those in charge of them. One can, therefore, only press the importance, as being yet greater in the case of children, greatest in the case of sick children, of attending to these things.

4   That which, however, above all, is known to injure children seriously is foul air, and most seriously at night. Keeping the rooms where they sleep tight shut up, is destruction to them. And, if the child's breathing be disordered by disease, a few hours only of such foul air may endanger its life, even where no inconvenience is left by grown-up persons in the same room.

5   The following passages, taken out of an excellent "Lecture on Sudden Death in Infancy and Childhood," just published, show the vital importance of careful nursing of children. "In the great majority of instances, when death suddenly befalls the infant or young child, it is an *accident;* it is not a necessary, inevitable result of any disease from which it is suffering."

6   It may be here added, that it would be very desirable to know how often death is, with adults, "not a necessary, inevitable result of any disease." Omit the word "sudden;" (for *sudden* death is comparatively rare in middle age;) and the sentence is almost equally true for

all ages.

7 The following causes of "accidental" death in sick children are enumerated:—"Sudden noises, which startle—a rapid change of temperature, which chills the surface, though only for a moment—a rude awakening from sleep—or even an over-hasty, or an over-full meal"—"any sudden impression on the nervous system—any hasty alteration of posture—in short, any cause whatever by which the respiratory process may be disturbed."

8 It may again be added, that, with very weak adult patients, these causes are also (not often "suddenly fatal," it is true, but) very much oftener than is at all generally known, irreparable in their consequences.

9 Both for children and for adults, both for sick and for well (although more certainly in the case of sick children than in any others), I would here again repeat, the most frequent and most fatal cause of all is sleeping, for even a few hours, much more for weeks and months, in foul air, a condition which, more than any other condition, disturbs the respiratory process, and tends to produce "accidental" death in desease.

10 I need hardly here repeat the warning against any confusion of ideas between cold and fresh air. You may chill a patient fatally without giving him fresh air at all. And you can quite well, nay, much better, give him fresh air without chilling him. This is the test of a good nurse.

11 In cases of long recurring faintnesses from diseases, for instance, especially disease which affects the organs of breathing, fresh air to the lungs, warmth to the surface, and often (as soon as the patient can swallow) hot drink, these are the right remedies and the only ones. Yet, oftener than not, you see the nurse or mother just reversing this; shutting up every cranny through which fresh air can enter, and leaving the body cold, or perhaps throwing a greater weight of clothes upon it, when already it is generating too little heat.

12 "Breathing carefully, anxiously, as though respiration were a function which required all the attention for its purpose," is cited as a not unusual state in children, and as one calling for care in all the things enumerated above. That breathing becomes an almost voluntary act, even in grown up patients who are very weak, must often have been remarked.

Conclusion

13. "Disease having interfered with the perfect accomplishment of the respiratory function, some sudden demand for its complete exercise, issues in the sudden stand still of the whole machinery," is given as one process:—"Life goes out for want of nervous power to keep the vital functions in activity," is given as another, by which "accidental" death is not often brought to pass in infancy.

14. Also in middle age, both these processes may be seen ending in death, although generally not suddenly. And I have seen, even in middle age, the *"sudden* stand-still" here mentioned, and from the same causes.

Summary.

15. To sum up :—the answer to two of the commonest objections urged, one by women themselves, the other by men, against the desirableness of sanitary knowledge for women, *plus* a caution, comprises the whole argument for the art of nursing.

Reckless amateur physicking by women. Real knowledge of the laws of health alone can check this.

16. (1.) It is often said by men, that it is unwise to teach women anything about these laws of health, because they will take to physicking, —that there is a great deal too much of amateur physicking as it is, which is indeed true. One eminent physician told me that he had known more calomel given, both at a pinch and for a continuance, by mothers, governesses, and nurses, to children than he had ever heard of a physician prescribing in all his experience. Another says, that women's only idea in medicine is calomel and aperients. This is undeniably too often the case. There is nothing ever seen in any professional practice like the reckless physicking by amateur females. Many ladies, having once obtained a "blue pill" prescription from a physician, will give and take it as a common aperient two or three times a week—with what effect may be supposed. The physician, being informed of it, substitutes for the prescription a comparatively harmless aperient pill. The lady complains that it "does not suit her half so well."

17. If women will take or give physic, by far the safest plan is to send for "the doctor" every time. There are those who both give and take physic, who will not take pains to learn the names of the commonest medicines, and confound, *e.g.,* colocynth with colchicum. This *is* playing with sharp-edged tools "with a vengeance."

18. There are also excellent women who will write to London to their physician that there is much sickness in their neighbourhood in the country, and ask for some prescription from him, which they "used

to like" themselves, and then give it to all their friends and to all their poorer neighbours who will take it. Now, instead of giving medicine, of which you cannot possibly know the exact and proper application, nor all its consequences, would it not be better if you were to persuade and help your poorer neighbours to remove the dung-hill from before the door, to put in a window which opens, or an Arnott's ventilator, or to cleanse and lime-wash their cottages? Of these things the benefits are sure. The benefits of the inexperienced administration of medicines are by no means so sure.

19 Homœopathy has introduced one essential amelioration in the practice of physic by amateur females; for its rules are excellent, its physicking comparatively harmless—the "globule" is the one grain of folly which appears to be necessary to make any good thing acceptable. Let then women, if they will give medicine, give homœopathic medicine. It won't do any harm.

20 An almost universal error among women is the supposition that everybody *must* have the bowels opened once in every twenty-four hours or must fly immediately to aperients. The reverse is the conclusion of experience.

21 This is a doctor's subject, and I will not enter more into it; but will simply repeat, do not go on taking or giving to your children your abominable "courses of aperients," without calling in the doctor.

22 It is very seldom indeed, that by choosing your diet, you cannot regulate your own bowels; and every woman may watch herself to know what kind of diet will do this; deficiency of meat produces constipation, quite as often as deficiency of vegetables; baker's bread much oftener than either. Home-made brown bread will oftener cure it than anything else.

23 A really experienced and observing nurse neither physics herself nor others. And to cultivate in things pertaining to health observation and experience in women who are mothers, governesses or nurses, is just the way to do away with amateur physicking, and if the doctors did but know it, to make the nurses obedient to them,—helps to them instead of hindrances. Such education in women would indeed diminish the doctor's work—but no one really believes that doctors wish that there should be more illness, in order to have more work.

24 (2.) It is often said by women, that they cannot know anything of the laws of health, or what to do to preserve their children's health,

What pathology teaches. What observation alone theaches. What medicine does. What nature alone does.

128   Conclusion

because they can know nothing of "Pathology," or cannot "dissect,"— a confusion of ideas which it is hard to attempt to disentangle. Pathology teaches the harm that disease has done. But it teaches nothing more. We know nothing of the principle of health, the positive of which pathology is the negative, except from observation and experience. And nothing but observation and experience will teach us the ways to maintain or to bring back the state of health. It is often thought that medicine is the curative process. It is no such thing; medicine is the surgery of functions, as surgery proper is that of limbs and organs. Neither can do anything but remove obstructions; neither can cure; nature alone cures. Surgery removes the bullet out of the limb, which is an obstruction to cure, but nature heals the wound. So it is with medicine; the function of an organ becomes obstructed; medicine, so far as we know, assists nature to remove the obstruction; but does nothing more. And what nursing has to do in either case, is to put the patient in the best condition for nature to act upon him. Generally, just the contrary is done. You think fresh air, and quiet and cleanliness extravagant, perhaps dangerous, luxuries, which should be given to the patient only when quite convenient, and medicine the *sine quâ non,* the panacea. If I have succeeded in any measure in dispelling this illusion, and in showing what true nursing is, and what it is not, my object will have been answered.

25   Now for the caution :—

What does *not* make a good nurse.

(3.) It seems a commonly received idea among men and even among women themselves that it requires nothing but a disappointment in love, the want of an object, a general disgust, or incapacity for other things, to turn a woman into a good nurse.

26   This reminds one of the parish where a stupid old man was set to be schoolmaster because he was "past keeping the pigs."

27   Apply the above receipt for making a good nurse to making a good servant. And the receipt will be found to fail.

28   Yet popular novelists of recent days have invented ladies disappointed in love or fresh out of the drawing-room turning into the war-hospitals to find their wounded lovers, and when found, forthwith abandoning their sick-ward for their lover, as might be expected. Yet in the estimation of the authors, these ladies were none the worse for that, but on the contrary were heroines of nursing.

29   What cruel mistakes are sometimes made by benevolent men and

women in matters of business about which they can know nothing and think they know a great deal.

30 The everyday management of a large ward, let alone of a hospital —the knowing what are the laws of life and death for men, and what the laws of health for wards—(and wards are healthy or unhealthy, mainly according to the knowledge or ignorance of the nurse)—are not these matters of sufficient importance and difficulty to require learning by experience and careful inquiry, just as much as any other art? They do not come by inspiration to the lady disappointed in love, nor to the poor workhouse drudge hard-up for a livelihood.

31 And terrible is the injury which has followed to the sick from such wild notions!

32 In this respect (and why is it so?), in Roman Catholic countries, both writers and workers are, in theory at least, far before ours. They would never think of such a beginning for a good working Superior or Sister of Charity. And many a Superior has refused to admit a *Postulant* who appeared to have no better "vocation" or reasons for offering herself than these.

33 It is true *we* make "no vows." But is a "vow" necessary to convince us that the true spirit for learning any art, most especially an act of charity, aright, is not a disgust to everything or something else? Do we really place the love of our kind (and of nursing, as one branch of it,) so low as this? What would the Mère Angélique of Port Royal, what would our own Mrs. Fry have said to this?

34 I would earnestly ask my sisters to keep clear of both the jargons now current everywhere (for they *are* equally jargons); of the jargon, namely, about the "rights" of women, which urges women to do all that men do, including the medical and other professions, merely because men do it, and without regard to whether this *is* the best that women can do; and of the jargon which urges woman to do nothing that men do, merely because they are women, and should be "recalled to a sense of their duty as women," and because "this is women's work," and "that is men's," and "these are thing which women should not do," which is all assertion and nothing more. Surely woman should bring the best she has, *whatever* that is, to the work of God's world, without attending to either of these cries. For what are they, both of them, the one *just* as much as the other, but listening to the "what people will say," to opinion, to the "voices from without?" And as a

The two jargons of the day.

wise man has said, no one has ever done anything great or useful by listening to the voices from without.

35   You do not want the effect of your good things to be, "How wonderful for a *woman!*" nor would you be deterred from good things, by hearing it said, "Yes, but she ought not to have done this, because it is not suitable for a woman." But you want to do the thing that is good, whether it is "suitable for a woman" or not.

36   It does not make a thing good, that it is remarkable that a woman should have been able to do it. Neither does it make a thing bad, which would have been good had a man done it, that it has been done by a woman.

37   Oh, leave these jargons, and go your way straight to God's work, in simplicity and singleness of heart.

SUPPLEMENTARY CHAPTER.

What is a Nurse?

1   This book takes away all the poetry of nursing, it will be said, and makes it the most prosaic of human things. My dear sister, there is nothing in the world, except perhaps education, so much the reverse of prosaic—or which requires so much power of throwing yourself into others' feelings which you have never felt,—and if you have none of this power, you had better let nursing alone. The very alphabet of a nurse is to be able to interpret every change which comes over a patient's countenance, without causing him the exertion of saying what he feels. What would many a nurse do otherwise than she does, if her patient were a valuable piece of furniture or a sick cow? I do not know. Yet a nurse must be something more than a lift or a broom. A patient is not merely a piece of furniture, to be kept clean and ranged against the wall, and saved from injury or breakage—though to judge from what many a nurse does and does not do you would say he was. But watch a good old-fashioned monthly nurse with the infant; she is firmly convinced, not only that she understands everything it "says," and that no one else can understand it, but also that it understands everything she says, and understands no one else.

2   Now a nurse *ought* to understand in the same way every change of her patient's face, every change of his attitude, every change of his

voice. And she ought to study them till she feels sure that no one else understands them so well. She may make mistakes, but she is *on the way* to being a good nurse. Whereas the nurse who never observes her patient's countenance at all, and never expects to see any variation, any more than if she had the charge of delicate china, is on the way to nothing at all. She never will be a nurse.

<small>Appearance of watching *not* good nursing.</small>

3 "He hates to be watched," is the excuse of every careless nurse. Very true. All sick people and all children "hate to be watched." But find a nurse who really knows and understands her children and her patients, and see whether these are aware that they have been "watched." It is not the staring at a patient which tells the really observant nurse the little things she ought to know. The best observer I know, a man whose labours among lunatics have earned for him the gratitude of Europe, appears to be quite absent. He leans back in his chair, with half-shut eyes, and, meanwhile, he sees everything, hears everything, observes everything; and you feel he knows you better than many who have lived with you twenty years. I believe it is this singular capacity of observation and of understanding what observed appearances imply, which gives him his singular influence over lunatics.

<small>What is experience?</small>

4 People often talk of a nurse who has been ten or fifteen years with the sick, as being an "experienced nurse." But it is observation only which makes experience; and a woman who does not observe might be fifty or sixty years with the sick and never be the wiser.

5 Nay more, experience sometimes tells in the opposite direction. "A man who practises the blunders of his predecessors," is often said to be "a practical man;" and she who perpetuates the "blunders of her predecessors" is often called an experienced nurse. The friends of a patient have been known to recommend the lodging in which he fell ill, just for the very reason which made him ill. A nurse has alleged as her reason for doing the things by which her predecessor ruined her own and her patient's health, that her predecessor "had always done them." People have taken a house because it had been emptied by death of all its occupants. These are they whom *no* experience will teach—viz., those who cannot see or understand the practical results of what they and others do. Now it is *no* reason that A did it for B to do it. It would be a reason if the results of A's doing it had been proved to be good.

6   What strikes one most with many women, who call themselves nurses, is that they have not learnt this A B C of a nurse's education. The A of a nurse ought to be to know what a sick human being is. The B to know how to behave to a sick human being. The C to know that her patient is a sick human being and not an animal.

7   What is it to feel a *calling* for any thing? Is it not to do your work in it to satisfy your own high idea of what is the *right*, the *best*, and not because you will be "found out" if you don't do it? This is the "enthusiasm" which every one, from a shoemaker to a sculptor, must have, in order to follow his "calling" properly. Now the nurse has to do, not with shoes, or with chisel and marble, but with human beings; and if she, for her own satisfaction, does not look after her patients, no *telling* will make her capable of doing so.

A nurse must feel a calling for her occupation.

8   A nurse who has such a "calling" will, for her own satisfaction and interest in her patient, inform herself as to the state of his pulse, which can be quite well done without disturbing him. She will have observed the state of the secretions, whether told to do so or not. Nay, the very appearance of them, a slight difference in colour, will betray to her observing eye that the utensil has not been emptied after each motion.

9   She will, in like manner, have observed the state of the skin, whether there is dryness or perspiration—the effect of the diet, of the medicines, the stimulants. And it is remarkable how often the doctor is deceived in private practice by not being told that the patient has just had his meal or his brandy. She will most carefully have watched any redness or soreness of the skin, always on her guard against bed sores. Any increasing emaciation will never come unknown to her. She will be well acquainted with the different eruptions of fevers, measles, &c., and premonitory symptoms. She will know the shiver which betrays the formation of matter—that which shows the unconscious patient's desire to pass water—that which precedes fever. She will observe the changes of animal heat in her patient, and whether periodical, and not consider him as a piece of inorganic matter, in keeping him warm or cool.

10   A nurse who has such a "calling" will look at all the medicine bottles delivered to her for her patients, smell each of them, and, if not satisfied, taste each. Nine hundred and ninety-nine times there will be no mistake, but the thousandth time there may be a serious

A nurse with a calling.

mistake detected by her means. But if she does not do this for her own satisfaction, it is no use telling her, because you may be sure that she will use neither smell nor taste to any purpose.

A nurse without the nurse's calling.

11 A nurse who has *not* such a "calling," will never be able to learn the sound of her patient's bell from that of others.

12 She will, when called to for hot brandy-and-water for her fainting patient, offer the weekly "Punch" (fact). Or she will wait to bring the cordial till she brings his tea (fact).

13 Under such a nurse, the patient never gets a hot drink. She pours out his tea, then she makes a journey to the larder for the butter, then she remembers that she has forgotten the toast, and has another journey to the kitchen fire to make the toast, then she fills a hot water bottle, and last of all she takes him his tea.

14 Such a nurse will never know whether her patient is awake or asleep. She will rouse him up to ask him "if he wants anything," and leave him uncared for when he *is* up.

15 She will make the room like an oven when he is feverish at night, and let out the fire when he is cold in the morning.

16 Such a nurse seems to have neither eyes, nor ears, nor hands.

17 She never touches any thing without a crash or an upset.

18 She does not shut the door, but pulls it after her, so that it always bursts open again.

19 She cannot rub in an embrocation without making a sore, which, in too many cases, never heals during the patient's life.

20 She catches up a cup and saucer in one hand, and pokes the fire with the other. Both of course come to "grief." Or she carries in a tray in one hand, and a coal scuttle in the other. Both of course tip out their contents. And she, in stooping to pick them up, knocks over the bedside table upon the patient with her head (fact).

21 Tables are made for things to stand upon—beds for patients to lie in.

22 But such a nurse puts down a heavy flower-pot upon the bed, or a large book or bolster which has rolled upon the floor.

23 Yet these things are not done by drinking Mrs. Gamps, but by respectable women, receiving their guinea a-week in private families.

A man's definition of a nurse.

24 Yet no *man,* not even a doctor, ever gives any other definition of what a nurse should be than this—"devoted and obedient."

25 This definition would do just as well for a porter. It might even

do for a horse. It would not do for a policeman. Consider how many women there are who have nothing to devote—neither intelligence, nor eyes, nor ears, nor hands. They will sit up all night by the patient, it is true; but their attendance is worth nothing to him, nor their observations to the doctor.

26   Cases have been known where the patient was cold before the nurse had observed he was dead—and yet she was not asleep—many cases where she supposed him comfortably sleeping, and he was insensible—very many where she never knew he was dying, unless he told her so himself.

27   But let no woman suppose that obedience to the doctor is not absolutely necessary. Only, neither doctor nor nurse lay sufficient stress upon *intelligent* obedience, upon the fact that obedience *alone* is a very poor thing.

28   I have known an obedient nurse told not to disturb a very sick patient as usual at ten o'clock with some customary service which she used to perform for him then, actually leave him in the dark all night, alleging this order as her reason for not carrying in his night light as usual.

29   Everybody has known the window left open in heavy fog or rain, or shut when the patient was fainting, by such obedient nurses.

30   There seems to be no medium for them between a furnace of a fire and no fire at all; and one is actually obliged in this variable climate to divide the year into two parts, and tell them—"Now no fire," "Now fire"; as if they were volunteer riflemen. You cannot trust them to make a *small* fire, although in England it is a question whether, except when the air without is hotter than the air within, patients are not always the better of some fire, if only to promote ventilation. But no; such nurses make it impossible.

31   Again, ladies generally give the definition of a good nurse as "sober, honest, and chaste." But would this not do for any other description of female service? Do you ask no more than this even from your cook or your housekeeper? *A lady's definition of a nurse.*

32   When you reflect how little, in England, women's powers of observation are exercised, how the prevailing impression is that almost any woman will do for a nurse, provided she is thus "sober" and "kind"—it seems most important that clinical instruction, so to speak, should be given to every nurse where alone it can be given,—in a

The elements of a nurse's duty.

33   The merest element of this is to call upon a nurse to observe the state of the pulse,—the effect of the diet,—of sleep, whether it has been distrubed,—whether there have been startings up in bed—a common mark of fatal disease, whether it has been a heavy, dull sleep, with stertorous breathing; whether there has been twitching of the bed-clothes,—to observe the state of the expectoration, the rusty expectoration of pneumonia, the frothy expectoration of pleurisy, the viscid mucous expectoration of bronchitis, the blood-streaked, dense, heavy expectoration which often occurs in consumption, —the nature of the cough itself by which the expectoration is expelled,—to observe the state of the secretions (yet nine-tenths of all nurses know nothing about these) whether the motions are costive or relaxed, and what is their colour, or whether there are alternations every few days of diarrhœa, and of no action of the bowels at all; whether the urine is high-coloured or pale, excessive, or scanty, muddy or clear, or whether it is high-coloured when the bowels do not act and pale when there is diarrhœa; whether there is ever blood in the motions, —in children, whether there are worms. All these things most nurses do not appear to consider it their business to observe.

34   The condition of the breathing and the position in which the patient breathes most easily, is another thing essential for the nurse to observe. In heart-complaints life is often extinguished by the patient "accidentally" falling into a position in which he cannot breathe—and life preserved by an "accidental" change of position. Now, what a thing it is to have to say of a nurse that it was not through her means, but through an "accident" that her patient was able to breathe.

35   Another essential duty of the nurse is, to observe the action of medicine;—as, for instance, that of quinine. The sore throat, the deafness, the tight feeling in the head, are well known effects of quinine. But the loss of memory it often occasions, is seldom known except to a very observant nurse. Indeed, she has often not memeory enough herself to remember that the patient has forgotten.

36   A good nurse scarcely ever asks a patient a question—neither as to what he feels nor as to what he wants. But she does not take for granted, either to herself or to others, that she knows what he feels and wants, without the most careful observation and testing of her own observations.

37 But why, for instance, should a nurse ask a private patient every day, "Please, sir, shall I bring your coffee?" or "your broth?" or whatever it is,—when she has every day brought it to him at that hour. One would think she did it for the sake of making the patient speak. Now, what the patient most wants is never to be called upon to speak about such things.

38 No sick man (in the *educated* classes) ever wishes for anything, in respect to his nurse, but that she should be as much out of the room as possible—a sufficient proof of what nursing *is now:* which, like other practical things, *is* always the consequence of what it is supposed it *ought to be.* A patient says, when his friends express uneasiness lest he should not be able to summon his nurse, "The last thing I should do, if I were worse, would be any thing to bring my nurse into the room, at least if I had my senses."

"Afraid of my nurse."

39 Such is nursing now. Amongst educated people, there is not one-half the fear of dying alone that there is of the nurse coming into the room.

40 There are a great many observations, of much importance, both physiologically and practically, which might be made by nurses, if they were educated to observation, and, indeed, can only be made by nurses or those who are always with the sick.

Observations which might be made by the sick bed.

41 I indicate them with the greatest diffidence, because of the little that is known upon them, and of my having no experience but my own to speak from.

42 Such are—

43 The different idea of time formed by the patient with the quick pulse and the patient with the slow pulse.

44 Dugald Stewart and other metaphysicians have speculated as to how we form our idea of time.

45 Without entering into any speculation, my experience is, that to the quick pulse the Arabian fables of a man putting his head under water, and the seconds appearing to him years, are all but realized.

46 A nurse's unpunctuality of ten minutes inflicts upon such a patient the idea of hours.

47 By the low, slow pulse, on the other hand, the lapse of time is almost unheeded.

48 Again, the physical difference of death-beds by different diseases,

138 Supplementary Chapter

is little observed. Patients who die of consumption very frequently die in a state of seraphic joy and peace; the countenance almost expresses rapture. Patients who die of cholera, peritonitis, &c., on the contrary, often die in a state approaching despair. The countenance expresses horror.

49   In dysentery, diarrhœa, or fever, the patient often dies in a state of indifference.

50   Again, in some cases, even of consumption and peritonitis, there are alternations almost of ecstacy and of despondency. In the lives of the "Saints," and in religious biographies we often find such deathbeds described truly enough. But then the patient and friends make unwise exertions to bring back the state of rapture, quite unaware that it may be only a physical state. And if it does not return, both may perhaps consider that its absence is a token of a state of "reprobation," or "backsliding."

51   Friends, in all these cases, are apt to judge most unfairly of the spiritual state of the sick from the physical manifestations.

52   Again, the question of temperaments is almost entirely unstudied in England for any practical purpose, except by medical men. And some patients are thought to suffer much less, some much more, than they really do. I have known a Celt rouse the whole hospital because his toes were cold. While, if an Anglo-Saxon said his back was cold, he was generally within 24 hours of death. An Anglo-Saxon man feels twice as much pain as he says; an Anglo-Saxon woman three times as much. You may generally believe half of what a Celtic man says he feels; and one-tenth of what a Celtic woman says.

53   Again, there are cases of disease of many classes and orders, which generate nervous power, without any balance of vital or digestive power, which is excessively misleading. The opposite case ceases to be able to produce brain power when the vital powers are exhausted. It falls asleep and eats. And its life is saved. But the first goes on able to think long after its powers of sleeping and eating are at an end, and neither patient himself nor others have any idea how ill he is. He dies simply because the powers of life go out.

54   These are two instances only of many varieties.

55   Again, there is a kind or stage of delirium which is often mistaken for dreaming, and *vice versâ.* Dreams almost always refer to times long ago. So does the low gentle delirium before death. I have known

great criminals talk of their mother's garden (like innocent children), just before death. And it has been supposed to be a sign of "grace."

56 Delirium and the visions produced by opium, generally refer to present things. The patient distorts what has very lately passed or just passed (or what is actually passing) around him, to his own imaginations.

57 I was once taken to see a great actress in Lady Macbeth. To me it appeared the mere transference upon the stage of a death-bed, such as I had often witnessed. So, just before death, have I seen a patient get out of bed, and feebly re-enact some scene of long ago, exactly as if walking in sleep.

58 There are many other physical observations, by which metaphysical questions might probably be solved. But it requires the world's accurate experience to gather data for them.

59 I only indicate a few.

Convalescence.

60 Many, indeed most, of the hints given for sickness will not do for convalescence; for instance, the *patient's* fancies about diet are often valuable indications to follow—the *convalescent's* often the reverse.

<small>Hints for the sick will not do for convalescents.</small>

61 Every nurse should make it a point to ascertain what are the signs of approaching convalescence. In all diseases these signs are more or less the same, but they are, or course, modified by the seat of the disease, as well as by its nature.

62 During disease, the system is engaged in throwing off dead or poisonous matters—during convalescence, in repairing waste. As soon as the vital powers have been freed there is a spring, as it were, towards health, operating irregularly, sometimes in the direction of one set of organs, sometimes of another. This is most remarkable in surgical injury, where there is fracture in more than one place. The patient distinctly feels like a set of little carpenters at work with little hammers, first at one fracture, then at another, never at both at once. Remark that a surgical patient *may*, and ought to be, in perfect health, during recovery from an accident—it is the fault of something else than the injury if he is not.

<small>Difference of sickness and convalescence.</small>

<small>Surgical patients should not be ill.</small>

63 When the diseased action has terminated, and convalescence has fairly set in, the patient very often has longings, especially for arti-

<small>Restraint necessary in convalescence.</small>

cles of food, which, if incautiously indulged, may lead to violent reaction, or even to relapse. The digestive functions are beginning to recover their power,—the most prominent symptom of which is increased appetite for food exceeding in quantity or quality (or both) what the stomach can digest. The utmost caution is necessary on the part of the nurse to prevent mischief from this cause. The medical attendant is, of course, the best judge of the food and regimen required; but during convalescence he is not there day by day, very often not above once or twice a week; and the nurse, at one of the most important periods of her patient's life, is left almost to herself —she has to be doctor and nurse too. It, therefore, very much depends upon her knowledge and experience whether the convalescence is to be slowly and steadily advanced, or whether it may not receive some rude check, throwing the patient back for weeks.

64 It has happened that a single well meant but ill-directed indulgence has ended in death.

Convalescent appetites.

65 In dieting convalescents, as a rule it is safer to keep *within* the patient's appetite than to satisfy it, and especially to go beyond it. Indeed, to satisfy the appetite of a convalescent is to go beyond what is required for nourishment, for the appetite is ahead of the power of digesting material to supply the waste occasioned by disease.

66 The nurse has often to deal not only with the patient's appetite, but with the officiousness of his friends. Some unwholesome, perhaps poisonous, delicacy is one of the first offerings generally made by them. The nurse should be on the watch against this—she ought to remember that her responsibility only ends when her services have been discontinued, and that she is really the person to see that the patient is dieted in strict conformity with the doctor's orders.

67 On the other hand, it may be that the main difficulty in the recovery is the patient's *want* of appetite, most likely to occur where he has no change of air. In such cases the nurse must exercise the same care in regard to diet and the times at which it is to be given, as is indicated for sickness at Chap. VI.

68 There are other indulgences besides those of the stomach which require to be kept under check. Some patients are apt to over-exert themselves in various ways, to incur unnecessary exposure and fatigue, perhaps to be followed by sitting in a draught. Friends often carry on long and exhausting conversations, or prolonged readings,

at one time, which are followed by a loss of vital power to the patient, requiring some time for its recovery. Errors in too much or too little clothing have also to be guarded against; but as a rule convalescents require warm clothing.

69   In all these things, a convalescent is, so to speak, like a child, neither mind nor body has recovered its proper tone, and, for a certain time differing in different diseases, the nurse has to guide him by her own experience. She has this great advantage, that she has watched the whole progress of the case, from the point of danger up to that of recovery, and by keeping the whole chain in view she will be able to find the right course.

70   It is not meant that she is to be like Sancho Panza's physician, and order every thing to be removed from table; she is there as before to exercise common sense and discretion. She must study her convalescent just as faithfully as she has studied her patient.

71   The activity and craving of the imagination, is like that of the stomach, extraordinary in some convalescents, especially in convalescents from fever. They have often an excessive craving for novels, not character novels, but melodramatic and incident novels. And if they cannot obtain such, they will, with singular lucidity of memeory and vigour of fancy, go over novels in their head which they have not read for twenty years. And they often state that never in their lives did they know what the pleasures of fancy were before. It is well not to let this go too far, as the terrors of some ghost story or appalling crime will have the same vividness in their imagination, and, creeping in unawares, become uncontrollable even to the degree of preventing sleep. *Convalescent imaginations.*

72   Change, a change of air, is of the very first importance as soon as the disease has "taken a turn." Every body must have remarked how a person recovering remains sometimes for weeks without making any progress, yet with apparently nothing the matter with him. The change from a ground-floor to an upstairs ward will sometimes hasten a patient's recovery. The mere move to what *he* considers the "convalescent" ward will give him a fillip. Change is essential. He must go to another place, or even only to another room. Then he immediately begins to "pick up." This is every day experience. But with the poor "change of air" is next to impossible. And people, without large experience, and who have never had a severe illness them- *Change of air essential.*

142 Supplementary Chapter

selves to enlighten them, have little idea how large a class there is (and for how long a time) who require an intermediate place between hospital and a convalescent Institution where there is *no* nursing. A place with the most careful nursing and every hospital comfort *together with country air* would save many lives from being spent in the Union Workhouse, many from requiring poor law relief at all, many from giving birth to unhealthy families, and many premature deaths.

<small>Convalescent institutions.</small> 73 There are those to whom this subject appears unimportant; such people say, when a sick man is convalescing, he is doing well, and there is an end of it. They never consider that convalescence has its degrees and its course the same as disease. And that you may have a very long convalescence instead of a short one, or perhaps no convalescence at all, by simply entertaining the habit of thought that "there is an end of it."

<small>Convalescents require nursing as well as country air.</small> 74 Such people do not see "why convalescents are to be *nursed* at all." And yet persons who have taken the pains to watch are perfectly well aware that many cases would be irretrievably lost but for careful nursing. Some would become permanent invalids; others burdens to themselves and their friends for the rest of their days. There may be return to *life;* but return to health and usefulness depends upon the *after-* nursing in almost all cases. Careful nursing has done in a few weeks what uncareful medical observation has declared it impossible to do in less than two years. Long convalescence ending in relapse or death is by no means unfrequent among the poor, many of whom leave hospital to make way for more necessitous cases long before they are able to return to their customary employment.

75 Follow these people to their homes, and what do you find? A straightened household, overtaxed to the utmost by a long illness of its head or support, receiving back, perhaps from expected death, its head (not to be a *support* but) to be a farther call upon its exhausted resources for nursing, clothing, and above all for suitable food and comforts. There can be no doubt that these defective convalescences, gone through in bad air and in the absence of almost every requisite, eventually go to swell the Registrar's Death List.

76 The question naturally arises, whether in contributing to a "County Hospital," one has done one's whole duty in this matter. Healthy people don't thrive very well if they sleep among sick people. Is it rational

to imagine that convalescents can do so either? Would it not appear a main point in regard to all hospitals in populous districts for each to have its convalescent branch at a convenient distance in the open country into which recovering cases should be drafted from the hospital wards as speedily as possible?

77 My own conviction is that, next to removing hospitals entirely out of towns, there is nothing which would add so much to the efficiency of these institutions, or, at the same time, be so great a blessing to the sick poor as henceforth to look on convalescence as a state as much requiring its special conditions and management as sickness; and to provide for it accordingly.

78 I rejoice to think that steps are being made in this direction both in London and Manchester.

Children in London.

79 It may be imagined that all these remarks apply only to the nursing of sick, whereas, in reality, there is another class, for whom they are equally important—and those are children—not sick, but "delicate," chiefly children of the richer classes, who, in spite of every care and no little expense, become a source of incessant anxiety to their parents, from excessive or from ignorant nursing.

To save not only the sick but "delicate" children—"delicate," owing to excessive nursing—chiefly in the class who can afford too much of everything artificial.

80 Many children who, during their stay in the country, are blooming in full vigour, are, during their town life, in an incredibly short time, transformed into delicate hot-house plants, for whose lives parents tremble after an hour's exposure to fresh air and cold. This is the result of their being transplanted into an artificial overtrained and over-nursed hot-house life, without having fresh air, or free exercise *ad libitum,* with altered diet, altered habits, coercion and restriction meeting them at every turn; and all this in badly constructed, badly ventilated, badly warmed houses, in a large town. All the good that has been built up during six months in the country, in a healthful life, is generally lost in one month of town life.

Not "London air" but London life does it.

Good gained in the country lost.

81 The popular belief is, that London air does it all; that children cannot thrive in it; and that all that is to be done is to keep them there for as short a time as possible.

82 But we forget the effect of the "air of London houses" and of London habits.

144 Supplementary Chapter

83   As to healthiness of site, there is a great difference between Hampstead, Camberwell, and Belgravia. The most densely populated and most filthy parts of a town are not the best neighbours to windward. The most elevated and exposed positions are generally the healthiest; the lowest to leeward of nuisances, under the shelter of the more elevated parts, generally the unhealthiest.

84   The low western districts, under the lee of London nuisances, are the recipients of foul air from the less healthy districts of London, whenever the wind comes from that direction; and yet people like to live there, because it is the "West End."

Difficult to poison a house in the country, in London very little will do it.

85   A house in the country isolated in healthy and pure air defies almost any amount of ignorance to make it unhealthy (and often one sees no little), but in the atmosphere of London very little indeed will do it.

Constant "smell of dinner" test.

86   Houses generally are not built to be ventilated. There is no way for the foul air to go out, and there is no way for fresh air to get in. The best popular test, because affecting everybody's senses, is the length of time which most houses retain the smell of dinner; some houses are seldom without it in the garrets. The only place whence the air of many a house is drawn is the basement and the kitchen.

87   The air both of basement and kitchen should be so pure as never to be offensive. Nothing offensive has any right to be there. Keep the air inside your house as pure as the air outside, by all means; a proper use of windows will enable you to do this, but never think of ventilation as a substitute for cleanliness.

Children in town go out (when they do) like dogs in leashes, or in a carriage.

88   But to return to children, how do they live in these houses? In the country they spend at least half their time in the open air; but in town, 99 hours out of 100 are spent in the house, and when they do go out, they go like dogs in leashes. This does away with all the healthy influence of play, of muscular exercise; there is not a run nor a laugh, nor a warm and red and healthy-looking face, and in many cases the delicate ones are packed up in a carriage to take the imaginary airing like a dose of medicine.

All this artificial fear not necessary, though it soon creates some foundation for itself.

89   Then that traditionary dread on the part of nurses of a "northeaster," which in their minds comprises about three-fourths of the compass. This dread is certainly justified when children have had a year's training as hot-house plants, which makes them like invalids after ten years' residence in the tropics, and which actually succeeds

in producing that educational monstrosity, rheumatic phthisicky invalids, of fifteen.

90   An amount of schooling which would be a fair allowance for twelve months is often condensed into a period of six or four months in London, on account of the greater facilities for tuition; at all events the "pupils" sit in the school-room, they sit in the drawing-room, they sleep in their bedroom or nursery, one closer than the other, one warmer than the other (sometimes they *sleep in warmed rooms*, the most injurious error in the regime of all young people), they do everything by order, everything according to rule, they become pale, lifeless shadows, in which there is no health, or strength, or spirit; nerves, muscles, and mind are all equally wanting in healthful exercise. *[Well-instructed lifeless victims.]*

91   I would add three other things, which exercise a terrible influence on the health of this class of children:— *[Three injuries to children.]*

92   1. I have seen people of large fortune exile their children (without the least scruple) to a north nursery (*qy.* nursery of scrofula), which never had one breath of sun-purified air; and these the most affectionate and anxious of parents.

93   2. The habit of having children "in to dessert." It is often said that this is the only time when a busy father can see his children. But, if there is "company," surely his seeing them then is not much good; and, if there is not, why must he see them over sweetmeats and wine?

94   3. I wonder whether many housekeepers' experience is the same as mine—viz., that in London houses "renewing" papers and furniture means putting a fresh paper a-top of a dirty one, and tacking a fresh chintz a-top of a dirty one,—aye, to *three* and four deep!! No wonder some London houses are always musty, if cleanliness has no more conscience than this! This clearly affects all the inmates; children only suffer in a greater degree.

95   The effects on the body are sometimes best tested by the state of appetite. Children who in the country have excellent appetites for animal, vegetable, and farinaceous food, for meat, milk, fruit, home-made bread, during their hothouse existence come down to bread and butter, tea, pastry, with an occasional orange. Is it a wonder that the stock should deteriorate under such "forcing?" *[Appetite-test; in country—in town.]*

96   Don't treat your children like sick—don't dose them with tea; *[Tea not to be given to children as to sick.]*

146 Supplementary Chapter

especially nervous and irritable children, who gain a little transient relief from it at the inevitable cost of their power of nutrition. Why not let them eat meat and drink half a glass of light beer, or milk? If they can't, rely upon it somebody is to blame, not the child nor the child's natural appetite.

Summary. 97 Give them fresh, light, sunny, and open schoolrooms, cool bedrooms, plenty of out-of-door exercise, facing even cold and wind and weather in sufficiently warm clothes and with sufficient exercise, plenty of amusement and play (free and according to the children's own schemes, not by order), more liberty and nature and less schooling and cramming and forcing and training; with more attention to food; less attention to physic—and you will find it possible to keep children in better health, even in the "air of London."

Note upon some Errors in Novels.

98 Novels do much to spread and stereotype popular errors and ignorances, forming, as they do now, so large a proportion of the reading of women of all classes. A few of the most common errors in novels are these:—

99 1. The joys of convalescence.—People must have had very different constitutions when they could rush back to life in the way recounted in fiction. In these days, for people of middle age, in the large towns of highly civilized communities, recovery (?) from severe illness is seldom recovery at all—is often delayed by relapse,—and is never anything but a struggle, slow and by no means "joyful." The assisting and encouraging, instead of overwhelming, convalescence is one of the most difficult and important duties of the nurse. Taking for granted that the patient is in a state of enjoyment, or even ease, is folly. Often, when he has no engrossing interest or affection, he is regretting the being called back to life which has then no zest for him. Or when these instantly re-seize their hold on him, he is making a painful effort to fulfil duties for which he feels himself totally unequal.

100 2. The loves of cousins are a favourite topic. The authors never think how they are assisting to thwart the plans of God for the human race.

101 3. Sick-beds and death-beds are painted with colours and des-

criptions which not only the novelist never could have seen, but which no one ever did see. There is perhaps but one novel-writer who is an exception to this.

102 In England, of all human experience, sickness and death have met with the least faithful observation. The materials of course are there, but the careful study is altogether wanting. The "death-bed" of almost every one of our novels is as mere a piece of stage-effect as is the singing-death of a prima donna in an opera. One would think death did not exist in reality. Shakespeare is the only author who has ever touched the subject with truth, and his truth is only on the side of art.

103 4. In novels, lives are saved by *"strong* jelly!" (what does *strong* jelly mean?) and by other things equally absurd.

104 5. The heroine always braves "contagion;" and then dies of it with her whole family or charge. More shame for her if they do!

105 Now, it is a question whether disease and death should be made matters of fiction at all. But if authors choose to write about such grave interests, surely it is not too much to ask that they will at least take the trouble to observe before they describe. Why should they encourage serious and even fatal mistakes? Why should they not inform themselves, for instance, as to what "infection" is, and make their heroine prevent it for others and herself, not partake in it, if such is to be the scene of her labours?

106 The true definition of infection is, that it is a means of spreading disease, which, when it exists, proves neglect or ignorance on the part of somebody, doctor, nurse, or relative; or that the place where it occurs is not fit for habitation, either by sick or by well.

Method of Polishing Floors.

107 [The object of this proceeding is only to obtain a good surface polish, in order to obviate the necessity of scrubbing. In all wood floors, except those of oak, a complete saturation, either with bees-wax or with *laque,* or with any indestructible material which may be thought better, so as to render the grain of the wood impervious, is the only thing perfectly safe for hospitals.]

108 Let the floors if not of oak be stained of that colour, but not too dark. No water should ever touch the boards after they are stained.

109 Bees-wax should be carefully prepared by scraping it into a vessel,

and covering it with spirits of turpentine; it should stand *covered over* until the wax is melted. It takes some hours to melt.

110   If the wax is dirty (as is often the case) melt it in the oven and then pour it carefully into another vessel leaving all sediment behind.

111   The wax should be only just soft enough to admit of its being well rubbed in, and off the boards.

112   Keep the softened wax always clean after it is made. If accidentally the polish becomes soiled, melt it again, and pour off the sediment as before. In applying it proceed as follows:—

1. Sweep the floor and wipe it clean from dust.
2. Spread the wax on the floor with discretion, *using very little.*
3. Take a soft thick cloth and rub it in well.
4. Take a second thick soft cloth and rub any superfluous wax off thoroughly.
5. If you use a polishing brush do so after this second cloth.
6. Then take a *soft duster* and polish, rubbing *briskly.* This process should be repeated twice a week.

113   N.B.—Be very careful to have your cloths *large* enough so that you may never have to rub twice with the same *dirty* piece, but always *fold* the cloth afresh as you go on.

114   Wash all the cloths after once using them. Do not wash the brush; put some turpentine into a plate, and rub the brush in it; pick out the little bits from it with a fork or stick. It should not require cleaning very often, if only used after the second cloth.

115   Floors if properly done, ought never to require bees-waxing more than twice a week. The high polish which the boards acquire repels dust and dirt.

116   A clean soft floor brush, and a clean soft cloth passed over once a day ought to remove all trace of dust.

117   This process does not require any additional labour or any more allowance of time than oft-repeated scouring. The boards once in good condition require no more labour than is expended in the ordinary ways by which rooms and wards are cleaned; with the additional benefit of being more healthy, and of saving patients exposure to damp exhalation from wet boards.

118   Before this plan was adopted floors of certain hospitals, owing to the constant passing and re-passing, had to be scrubbed every day. The stained boards have stood the test of seven years' experience,

and they have been kept in order by women and girls at the same amount of time which they before bestowed upon the scrubbing system.

Note upon Employment of Women.

119   People have written of late years immensely upon the non-"market" for "female labour," the want of "demand," or of "field," for the "industrial" employment of "women." My experience is, that the "demand" is many times greater than the *supply,* that the market for "female labour" is large, but the *labourers* are few. I limit myself to my own personal experience and particular field, and of course to paid labour. I do not avail myself of information collected as to other employments, such as that of teachers, both in families and in national schools, in which experience is the same as mine is in nursing. As to nursing, then, I have had, during the last three years, several hundreds of applications to recommend qualified matrons or superintendents of institutions—qualified missionary or parish nurses (*i.e.,* to nurse in a parish with a salary, derived not from Boards of Guardians but from proprietors in the parish)—qualified sick nurses for private families, for hospitals, and workhouses. Now, in all this the lack was of qualified nurses to fill the places, not of places for the nurses, had they existed, to fill. At a rough guess, I should say that about one-third of these applicants offered ample remuneration; another third fixed no rate but were willing to enter into any agreement suitable to the qualifications of the nurse; and the remaining third, (principally workhouses and provincial hospitals), offered a sum which could not have obtained the qualifications they required in any case.

120   I can only re-echo, as to nurses, what *Fraser* says as to "national school teachers," that "the demand" "at this moment far exceeds the supply of qualified persons."

121   If all the crowd of female writers who have enlarged on the employment of women, on women's just right to a field, and to adequate pay for their labour, were each to train (or to put into the way of training), ten women to supply the demand which is *already* open, we can hardly hesitate as to what the superiority of the result would be.

122   I am permitted to say by a friend who has (instead of writing about) tried it upon her own premises, in the matter of *female printers,*

150 Supplemenatry Chapter

that the experiment has fully succeeded, that the women earn good and even high wages (from 15*s*. to 25*s*. per week), that they do not work long hours, but have time over for domestic employment, and still the enterprise pays itself.

Note as to the Number of Women Employed as
Nurses in Great Britain.

123   25,466 were returned, at the census of 1851, as nurses by profession, 39,139 nurses in domestic service,* and 2,822 midwives. The numbers of different ages are shown in Table A, and in Table B their distribution over Great Britain.

124   To increase the efficiency of this class, and to make as many of them as possible the disciples of the true doctrines of health, would be a great national work.

125   For there the material exists, and will be used for nursing, whether the real "conclusion of the matter" be to nurse or to poison the sick. A man, who stands perhaps at the head of our medical profession, once said to me, "I send a nurse into a private family to nurse my Patient, but I know that the result is only to do him harm."

126   Now a nurse means any person in charge of the personal health of another. And, in the preceding notes, the term *nurse* is used indiscriminately for amateur and professional nurses. For, besides nurses of the sick and nurses of children, the numbers of whom are here given, there are friends or relations who take temporary charge of a sick person, there are mothers of families. It appears as if these unprofessional nurses were just as much in want of knowledge of the laws of health as professional ones.

127   Then there are the school-mistresses of all national and other schools throughout the kingdom. How many of children's epidemics originate in these! Then the proportion of girls in these schools, who become mothers or members among the 64,600 nurses recorded above, or schoolmistresses in their turn. If the laws of health, as far as regards fresh air, cleanliness, light, &c., were taught to these, would this not prevent some children being killed, some evil being

(119)   * A curious fact will be shown by Table A, viz., that 18,122 out of 39,139, or nearly one-half of all the nurses, in domestic service, are between 5 and 20 years of age; "while of public or professional nurses, about the same proportion are over sixty years of age."

perpetuated? On women we must depend, first and last, for personal and household hygiene—for preventing the family from degenerating in as far as these things are concerned. Would not the true way of infusing the art of preserving its own health into the human race be to teach the female part of it in schools and hospitals, both by practical teaching and by simple experiments, in as far as these illustrate what may be called the theory of it?

APPENDIX

Minding Baby

1. And now, girls, I have a word for you. You and I have all had a great deal to do with "minding baby," though "baby" was not our own baby. And we would all of us do a great deal for baby, which we would not do for ourselves.

2. Now, all that I have said about nursing grown-up people applies a great deal more to nursing baby. For instance, baby will suffer from a close room when you don't feel that it is close. If baby sleeps even for a few hours, much more if it is for nights and nights—in foul air, baby will, without any doubt whatever, be puny and sickly, and most likely to have measles or scarlatina, and not get through it well.

3. Baby will feel want of fresh air more than you. Baby will feel cold much sooner than you. Above all, baby will suffer more from not being kept clean (only see how it enjoys being washed in nice luke-warm water). Baby will want its clothes and its bed-clothes changed oftener than you. Baby will suffer more from a dirty house than you. Baby must have a cot to itself; else it runs the risk of being over-laid or suffocated. Baby *must* not be covered up too much in bed, nor too little. The same when it is up. And you must look after these things. Mother is perhaps too busy to see whether baby is too much muffled up or too little.

4. You must take care that baby is not startled by loud sudden noises; all the more you must not wake it in this way out of its sleep. Noises which would not frighten you, frighten baby.

5. And many a sick baby has been killed in this way.

6. You must be very careful about its food; about being strict to the minute for feeding it; not giving it too much at a time (if baby is sick after its food, you *have* given it too much). Neither must it be under-fed. Above all, never give it any unwholesome food, nor anything at

all to make it sleep, unless the doctor orders it.

7   If you knew how many, even well-to-do, babies I have known who have died from having had something given to make them sleep, and "keep them quiet"—not the first time, nor the second, nor the tenth time, perhaps—but at last.

8   I could tell you many true stories, which have all happened within my own knowledge, of mischief to babies from their nurse neglecting these things.

9   Here are a few:

10   1. Baby, who is weaned, requires to be fed often, regularly, and not too much at a time.

11   I know a mother whose baby was in great danger one day from convulsions. It was about a year old. She said she had wished to go to church; and so, before going, had given it its three meals in one. Was it any wonder that the poor little thing had convulsions?

12   I have known (in Scotland) a little girl, not more than five years old, whose mother had to go great distances every day, and who was trusted to feed and take care of her little brother, under a year old. And she always did it right. She always did what mother told her. A stranger coming into the hut one day (it was no better than a hut) said: "You will burn baby's mouth." "Oh, no," she said, "I always burn my own mouth first."

13   2. When I say, be careful of baby, I don't mean have it always in your arms. If the baby is old enough, and the weather warm enough for it to have some heat in itself, it is much better for a child to be crawling about than to be always in its little nurse's arms. And it is much better for it to amuse itself than to have her always making noises to it.

14   The healthiest, happiest, liveliest, most beautiful baby I ever saw was the only child of a busy laundress. She washed all day in a room with the door open upon a larger room, where she put the child. It sat or crawled upon the floor all day, with no other play-fellow than a kitten, which it used to hug. Its mother kept it beautifully clean, and fed it with perfect regularity. The child was never frightened at anything. The room where it sat was the house-place; and it always gave notice to its mother when anybody came in, not by a cry, but by a crow. I lived for many months within hearing of that child, and never heard it cry day or night.

15   I think there is a great deal too much of amusing children now; and not enough of letting them amuse themselves.

16   Never distract a child's attention. If it is looking at one thing, don't show it another; and so on.

17   3. At the same time, dullness and especially want of light, is worse for children than it is for you.

18   A child was once brought up quite alone in a dark room, by persons who wished to conceal its being alive. It never saw any one, except when it was fed; and though it was treated perfectly kindly, it grew up an idiot. This you will easily guess.

19   Plenty of light, and sunlight particularly, is necessary to make a child active, and merry, and clever. But, of all things, don't burn baby's brains out by letting the sun bake its head when out, especially in its little cart, on a hot summer's day.

20   *Never* leave a child in the dark; and let the room it lives in be *always* as light as possible, and as sunny. Except, of course, when the doctor tells you to darken the room, which he will do in some children's illnesses.

21   4. Do you know that one-half of all the nurses in service are girls of from five to twenty years old? You see, you are very important little people. Then there are all the girls who are nursing mother's baby at home; and, in all these cases, it seems pretty nearly to come to this, that baby's health for its whole life depends upon you, girls, more than upon anything else.

22   I need hardly say to you, what a charge! For I believe that you, all of you, or nearly all, care about baby too much not to feel this nearly as much as I do. You, all of you, want to make baby grow up well and happy, if you knew how.

23   So I say again:

24   5. The main want of baby is always to have fresh air.

25   You can make baby ill by keeping the room where it sleeps tight shut up, even for a few hours.

26   You can kill baby when it *is* ill by keeping it in a hot room, with several people in it, and all the doors and windows shut.

27   The doctor who looks after the Queen's children says so.

28   This is the case most particularly when the child has something the matter with its lungs and its breathing.

29   I found a poor child dying in a small room, tight shut up, with a

large fire, and four or five people round it to see it die. Its breathing was short and hurried; and it could not cough up what was choking its lungs and throat—mucus it is called. The doctor, who was a very clever man, came in, set open door and window, turned everybody out but one, and stayed two hours to keep the room clear and fresh. He gave the child no medicine; and it was cured simply by his fresh air.

30   A few hours will do for baby, both in killing and curing it, what days will not do for a grown-up person.

31   Another doctor found a child (it was a rich one) dying in a splendid close room, nearly breathless from throat complaint. He walked straight to the window and pulled it open; "for," he said, "when people can breathe very little air, they want that little good." The mother said he would kill the child. But, on the contrary, the child recovered.

32   But—

33   6. Take you care not to let a draught blow upon a child, especially a sick child.

34   Perhaps you will say to me: "I don't know what you would have me do. You puzzle me so. You tell me, don't feed the child too much, and don't feed it too little; don't keep the room shut up, and don't let there be a draught; don't let the child be dull, and don't amuse it too much." Dear little nurse, you must learn to *manage*. Some people never do learn management. I have felt all these difficulties myself; and I can tell you that it is not from reading my book that you will learn to mind baby well, but from practising yourself how best to manage to do what other good nurses (and my book, if you like it) tell you.

35   But about the draughts.

36   It is all nonsense what some old nurses say, that you can't give baby fresh air without giving it a chill; and, on the other hand, you may give baby a chill which will kill it (by letting a draught blow upon it when it is being washed, for instance, and chilling its whole body, though only for a moment), without giving it fresh air at all; and depend upon this, the less fresh air you give to its lungs, and the less water you give to its skin, the more liable it will be to cold and chills.

37   If you can keep baby's air always fresh indoors and out of doors,

and never chill baby, you are a good nurse.

38   A sick baby's skin is often cold, even when the room is quite close. Then you must air the room, and put hot flannels or hot bottles (not too hot) next baby's body; and give it its warm food.

39   But I have often seen nurses doing just the contrary, namely, shutting up every chink and throwing a great weight of bedclothes over the child, which makes it colder, as it has no heat in itself.

40   You would just kill a feverish child by doing this.

41   A children's doctor, very famous in London, says that when a sick child dies, it is just as often an *accident* as not; that is, people kill it by some foolish act of this kind, just as much as if they threw it out of a window. And he says, too, that when a sick child dies suddenly, it is almost always an accident. It might have been prevented. It was not that the child was ill, and so its death could not be helped, as people say.

42   He tells us what brings on these sudden deaths in sick children: Startling noises; chilling the child's body; wakening it suddenly; feeding it too much or too quickly; altering its posture suddenly, or shaking it roughly; frightening it. And to this you may add (more than anything else, too), *keeping it in foul air, especially when asleep, especially at night,* even for a few hours, and even when you don't feel it yourself. This is, most of all, what kills babies.

43   Baby's breathing is so tender, so easily put out of order. Sometimes you see a sick baby who seems to be obliged to attend to every breath it draws, and to "breathe carefully," in order to breathe at all; and if you disturb it rudely, it is all over with baby. Anything which calls upon it for breath may stop it altogether.

44   7. *Remember to keep baby clean.* I can remember when mothers boasted that *their* "children's feet had never been touched by water; no, nor any part of them but faces and hands"; that somebody's "child had had its feet washed, and it never lived to grow up," etc.

45   But we know better now. And I daresay you know that to keep every spot of baby's body always clean, and never to let any pore of its tender skin be stopped up by dirt or unwashed perspiration is the only way to keep baby happy and well.

46   It is a great deal of trouble; but it is a great deal more trouble to have baby sick.

47   The safest thing is to wash baby all over once or twice a day;

and to wash it besides whenever it has had an accidental wetting. You know how easily its tender skin gets chafed.

48   There may be a danger in washing a child's feet and legs only. There never can be in washing it all over. Its clothes should be changed oftener than yours, because of the greater quantity baby perspires. If you clothe baby in filth, what can you expect but that it will be ill? Its clothes must never be tight, but light and warm. Baby if not properly clothed, feels sudden changes in the weather much more than you do. Baby's bed-clothes must be clean oftener than yours.

49   Now, can you remember the things you have to mind for baby? There is—
   1. Fresh air.
   2. Proper warmth.
   3. Cleanliness for its little body, its clothes, its bed, its room, and house.
   4. Feeding it with proper food, at regular times.
   5. Not startling it or shaking either its little body or its little nerves.
   6. Light and cheerfulness.
   7. Proper clothes in bed and up.

50   And **management** in *all* these things.

51   I would add **one** thing. It is as easy to put out a sick baby's life as it is to put out the flame of a candle. Ten minutes' delay in giving it food may make the difference.

解 説
Interpretation

　本書にはフロレンス・ナイチンゲールの Notes on Nursing（「看護覚え書」）の全文を収める。これはナイチンゲールの代表的な著作であり、また看護にとってもっとも重要な古典であるといわれている。この本の初版は1859年の12月に出版されたが、たちまちのうちに英国中でベストセラーとなり、看護婦はもとより、一般市民からヴィクトリア女王にいたる人々が感激をもって読んだと伝えられている。

　この本の序でナイチンゲールが述べているように、もともとこれは看護の教科書として書かれたものではなく、一般市民とくに女性に向けて書かれたものであった。しかしこの本は出版されて以来長期間にわたって看護学校のテキストとして用いられてきたのであるが、その理由は、看護とは何をすることかという問いに対して、これほど見事にまたこれほど完璧に答えている書物が他にないからであり、かつまたナイチンゲールがここに、時代の変遷や文明の相違などにかかわりなく常に正しい看護のあり方の本質を述べているからであろう。

　文章は一見したところ平凡な内容しかないようにみえるし、ごく当り前のことを述べているにすぎないと思われるかもしれない。しかし、深く読みこんで行くと、その底には驚嘆すべきナイチンゲールのものの認識の仕方あるいは生命観が秘められていることが判ってくる。それは実は看護というはたらきそのものの性質に由来するものであろう。すなわち、看護は一見したところ平凡な何でもないはたらきのように見えて、その実、その底に生命の深奥に迫る英知を秘めているからであろう。

　全体は次のような構成になっている。
　　序
　　前文
　⑴　換気と暖房
　⑵　家屋の健康
　⑶　小管理
　⑷　騒音
　⑸　変化
　⑹　食事
　⑺　食物
　⑻　ベッドと寝具類
　⑼　光
　⑽　部屋と壁の清潔
　⑾　からだの清潔
　⑿　元気づけと助言
　⒀　病人の観察
　　結語
　　補章
　　付録・赤ん坊の世話

　なお、原著には目次の次に digest が入っており、また本文の欄外には小見出しが付せられているが、本書では省略した。

　ナイチンゲールは、初版発行以来何回かにわたって、この本に改訂を加えて出版しているので、現在この本は数種類の版本として残っている。本書では1860年増補改訂新版（ new edtion, revised and enlarged 1860. ）を採用し、それに1861年版労働者階級のための看護覚え書（Notes on Nursing for the Labouring Classes. 1861 ）の付録 "Minding Baby" を付すことにした。現在出版されている Notes on Nursing（原文）は数種類あり、そのほと

159

んどが1859年初版あるいは1861年労働者階級版をとっているが、これらには1860年増補改訂新版の **Supplementary Chapter** が付いていない。本書ではこの **Supplementary Chapter** の重要性にかんがみ、あえて1860年増補改訂新版を採ることにした。

(小南　吉彦)

First edition, July 1974 ©
Second edition, May 2001 ©

Florence Nightingale
NOTES ON NURSING

Compiled by
Hiroko Usui/Yoshihiko Kominami

Gendaisha Publishing Co., Ltd
Tokyo

〈原文看護学選集1〉 原文 看護覚え書

1974年 7月15日	第1版第1刷発行 ©
2001年 5月30日	第2版第1刷発行 ©
2016年 1月15日	第2版第5刷発行

編者代表　薄井坦子
発行者　小南吉彦

検印廃止

印刷　中央印刷株式会社
製本　誠製本株式会社

発行所　東京都新宿区早稲田鶴巻町514　株式会社 現代社
電話 03(3203)5061　振替 00150-3-68248

＊落丁本乱丁本はお取り替えいたします。

ISBN 978-4-87474-104-7

フロレンス・ナイチンゲールの生涯（全二巻）

C.ウーダム=スミス著　武山満智子他訳

第1版　1981年　Ａ5判　上製本　ケース入　各巻420頁　揃価5,600円
（税別）

　フロレンス・ナイチンゲールの伝記といえば，わが国ではこれまで少年少女向けの，いわば偉人伝的なものあるいは簡略なものしか紹介されてこなかった。したがって，彼女の真の姿や詳細な足跡を知り，さらに彼女の著作を深く理解しようとする者にとっては，納得のいく資料は皆無であったといっても過言ではない。本書はその意味からも出版を待ち望まれていた，英国の歴史作家ウーダム=スミス女史の700頁におよぶ大作"Florence Nightingale"の完訳である。

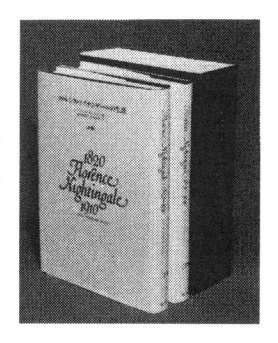

　これまで世に出されたナイチンゲールの詳細な伝記としては，他にＥ．クック卿のものが著名であるが，時代の制約や諸々の事情から彼の伝記には，かなりの重要な事実や書簡が欠けており，史実の叙述に物足りなさを感じることは否めなかった。しかし，スミス女史は，これらナイチンゲールの生涯を語るにはなくてはならない書簡や資料を適宜収載し，綿密な筆運びで，近代看護の先駆者の姿をあますところなく再現したのである。ここに初めてナイチンゲールの言葉が，そしてその真の生涯が時代を超えて鮮やかに蘇る。

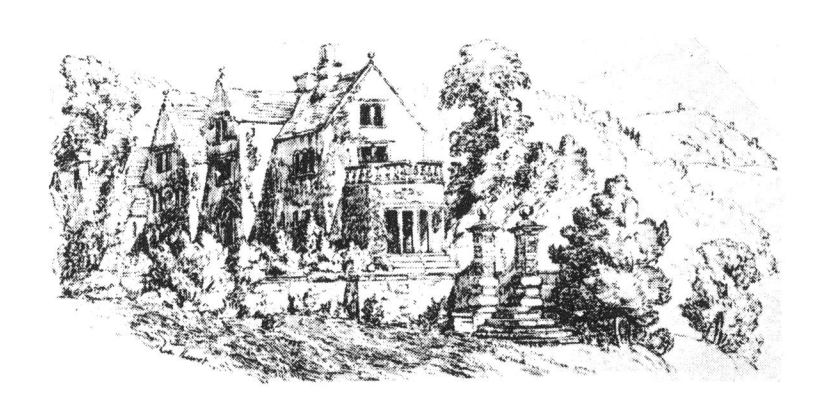

日本翻訳文化賞・日本翻訳出版文化賞 受賞

ナイチンゲール著作集（全三巻）

F.ナイチンゲール著　湯槇ます監修・薄井坦子他訳

第一巻＝第2版　1983年　Ａ５判　上製本　ケース入　520頁　3,800円
第二巻＝第1版　1974年　Ａ５判　上製本　ケース入　392頁　3,400円
第三巻＝第1版　1977年　Ａ５判　上製本　ケース入　532頁　3,900円
（税別）

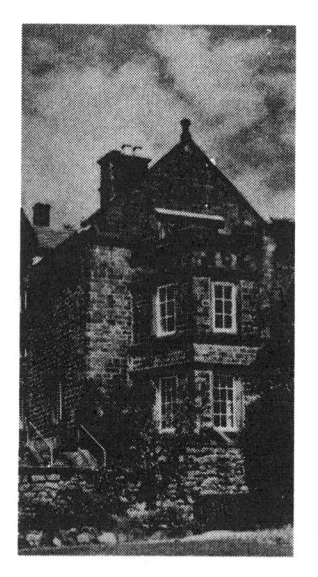

第一巻
　カイゼルスウエルト学園によせて　1851年
　女性による陸軍病院の看護　1858年
　看護覚え書——第４版増補改訂版　1860年
　インドの病院における看護　1865年
　　（付）ナイチンゲール著作目録

第二巻
　救貧院病院における看護　1867年
　貧しい病人のための看護　1876年
　病院と患者　1880年
　看護婦の訓練と病人の看護　1882年
　病人の看護と健康を守る看護　1893年
　町や村での健康教育——農村の衛生　1894年
　病院覚え書——第３版増補改訂版　1863年
　　（付）ナイチンゲール関係年表

第三巻
　インド駐在陸軍の衛生　1863年
　インドにおける生と死　1874年
　思索への思唆（抄）　1860年
　アグネス・ジョーンズをしのんで　1871年
　看護婦と見習生への書簡（14篇）　1872年～1900年
　　（付）ナイチンゲールに関する文献目録

　人類の歴史に不朽の業績を残しながら，この百年間，とかく曲解されることのみ多かったフロレンス・ナイチンゲールの，その生涯と思想とを知る手がかりとして，代表的な著作を集めて翻訳出版された待望の書。
　これほど世界にあまねくその名を知られたナイチンゲールでありながら，かつてわれわれは一度でも，彼女自身の手になる著作を翻いたことがあっただろうか。本著作集は，現在ではほとんど入手不可能といわれる，約150篇の彼女の全著作の中から30篇を選んで編訳上梓したものであるが，ここにはじめて思想家としてのナイチンゲールの「生命哲学」と「看護の思想」の全貌が明らかにされた。
　世界中に健康の危機が迫りつつある今日において，この生命哲学は強烈で新鮮な響きを増してきている。ひとり看護や医療に携わる者のみならず，汎く人間生命を究めんとする人々にとって必読の書である。

> ### ナイチンゲールの再認識
>
> 　　監修者のことば————————湯槇　ます
>
> 　私がフロレンス・ナイチンゲールの生涯と仕事の意味を改めて考え直してみるようになったのは，そんなに遠い日のことではない。（略）
> 　かねてより近代看護はナイチンゲールから始まると言いながら，ほんとにその意味を私が実感したのはこの頃のことなのである。世界中に健康の危険が迫って来たと言われる今日，ナイチンゲールの看護の思想にあらためて触れることは強烈で新鮮であった。「看護とは何か」の大きな方向が百年前にすでに示されていると発見し驚いたのである。また彼女の悲観しない現実的な精神に触れて心をうたれる。（略）
> 　ナイチンゲールの思想をあらためて確認しようとした私は，わが国に紹介されている彼女の著作が非常に少ないことに気がついた。ごくわずかしか資料がないのにナイチンゲールを知っていると思っているのは錯覚ではないだろうか。ナイチンゲールをもっとよく知りたいという思いは，その著作をできるだけたくさん読みたいという願いになった。
> 　ナイチンゲールの著作を読み訳出するには，看護を深く究めていること，彼女の幅広くかつ深い教養を消化できることが必要であると思う。ここに数名の者が集まってその訳業を始めた。訳出の仕事をする資格のいずれにおいても未熟であるのを充分承知しながら，あえて私たちがその役割をとったのは，「看護とは何か」の汲みつくせぬ答を含んでいる一連の著作を一日も早く，多くの人々に直接読んでいただきたいと願うからである。またこれにより看護という貴重な活動がさらに豊かにならんことを願うのである。
> 　　　　　　　　　　　　　　　　　　　　　　　（本書第二巻　月報より）

覆刻版 看護覚え書（品切）

F.ナイチンゲール著
1980年　キク変型　上製本　函入　242頁　8,000円
（税別）

　これは Florence Nightingale. Notes on Nursing, 2nd edition, revised and enlarged, 1860（看護覚え書，増補改訂2版）の完全覆刻版である。
　現在，Notes on Nursing の 1st edition は英国などにおいて覆刻されており，入手可能であるが，より資料的価値の高いとされているこの 2nd edition は，いままで覆刻されることなく，その原本はほとんど入手不可能であった。
　今回小社では，幸いにして1860年版の貴重な原本を入手することができたのを機会に，本書の完全覆刻に踏み切った。
　ひとりナイチンゲール研究家のみならず，看護に携わる方すべてにとって，得難い貴重本の1,000部限定，愛蔵版である。